SPEEDBUMPS

● ● ● ● ●

LIVING LIFE WITH EPILEPSY

SPEEDBUMPS
LIVING LIFE WITH EPILEPSY

JONATHAN B. DODSON WITH ELLEN WEISS DODSON

ILLUSTRATIONS BY TERRY DODSON

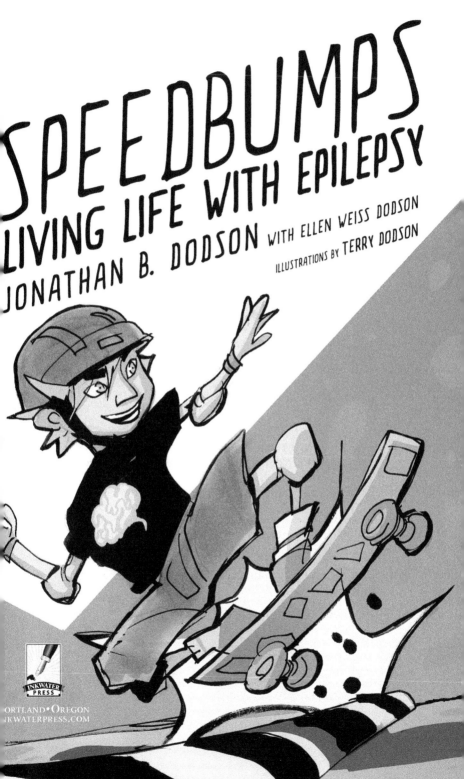

INKWATER
PRESS

PORTLAND • OREGON
INKWATERPRESS.COM

Publisher: Inkwater Press | www.inkwaterpress.com

Paperback ISBN-13 978-1-62901-611-5 | ISBN-10 1-62901-611-X
Kindle ISBN-13 978-1-62901-612-2 | ISBN-10 1-62901-612-8

1 3 5 7 9 10 8 6 4 2

To Dr. Elizabeth, who believed.
To my mom, who always knew.
To my dad, who has infinite patience.
To my wife, who loves me the way I am.
To my son, who is my greatest hope.

CONTENTS

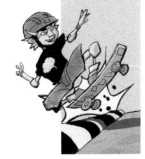

Fire all of your guns at once
And explode into space

"Born to be Wild" – Steppenwolf

A Mother's Message

A mother knows her child better than anyone.

I knew from an extremely young age that my son, Jonathan, was experiencing seizures. He started life as a brilliant child—early to walk, early to read. He was sociable and verbal in the most joyous ways. He slept through the night, had the typical bouts of ear infection and strep throat. He loved to count, sing the alphabet song, and eat fish sticks. Then one day I thought I detected a barely perceptible movement in his eyes—a slight rolling upward into his lids. I cannot tell you whether, in that moment, this was the first time it had happened, or if he had been doing it for months, but on that day I made a mental note of it. After that, this quirky eye roll happened with greater and greater frequency. If he was speaking when it occurred, it might seem only as if his breath hitched. He never froze, stared, or lost his train of thought.

But there it was—an anomaly so slight that you could have ignored it, had it not repeated with such regularity. He was then just twenty-two months old.

My husband and I both had big careers. As a working mom and dad, we sent our son to daycare out of practical necessity. We spent a lot of effort selecting a diverse, stimulating, and caring environment for our active little boy. Despite the long day he spent away from home, we nonetheless were able to cram a lot of activities into the short period between 6:00 p.m. and bedtime. My job required that I travel frequently, leaving much of the post-daycare duties to my husband. Although my husband could be deliberately clumsy at chores he disliked, such as fixing dinner or sorting laundry, he excelled at playtime and bath time with our young son—a "mini-me" of his very own. As man and man-child they were thick as thieves. It was not uncommon that I returned home from a business trip only to discover that my son had learned a few new "guy tricks," such as blowing bubbles through a straw into his milk, or swallowing air only to belch it up unapologetically on command.

Parenthood was our happy place. It made the stress of our jobs disappear. At that tender and innocent age, children are the very best source of entertainment. We loved reading together or building with Legos far more than answering emails or watching the latest episode of the *The X-Files*. No alien invasion offered more excitement than our own little life form, his every sound and movement a revelation to us as first-time parents.

I was one of *those* kind of parents, always waving a new set of photos straight from the lab. Just ask my former co-workers how they tired of being ambushed at the Coke machine with the latest shots of boy-on-blanket, boy-on-swing, boy-with-food-on-face, or boy-with-football jersey.

But as joyous as new parenthood could be, it came accompanied with abject fear. I continually monitored and double-checked everything. I could not help the compulsion to scrutinize with my maternal X-ray eyes, obsessing over every freckle and hair, scratch and bump. Despite my husband's and my successful accomplishments as professionals, we could not help but be clumsy parents, as we were truly powerless to protect our defenseless little ones from every lurking danger.

After I first observed my son's little eye effect I began keeping track of how frequently it occurred. It was most perceptible when he was the center of attention—reading aloud, singing, or talking. While it became more and more obvious to me, most people did not pick up his eye movement or associate it with the disruption in his speech pattern that was beginning to emerge, a sort of hiccup between his rapid-fire words. It was only a split second here and there and was easy to miss. I did not want to be perceived as a crazy, obsessed mother. I worked up the nerve to discreetly ask the teacher at daycare to observe my son closely. At the end of the day she had nothing unusual to report. Nonetheless, I continued to see his eyes roll, sometimes several times each hour. I shared my concerns with my husband, who is a doctor, that I thought there was an issue with our son. It took many months before he acknowledged seeing what I had been seeing. From a medical standpoint he thought it was unremarkable, describing it as a "reboot" or a skipped beat. He concluded that this "tic" was just an artifact of an active, precocious kid who was trying to say and do so many things at once.

Then the scariest moment happened. It was Easter Sunday and we were having dinner with our little family. There were four of us now, as our baby daughter had joined the mix. Jonathan, who was now nearly four, was entertaining us with his usual childish banter when his head fell, suddenly and aimlessly, toward his plate. He recovered just before connecting with his mashed potatoes, pulling his head upright and continuing his sentence right where he had left off. This was the first time that any physical effect manifested beyond the rolling of his eyes. I was horrified. Fortunately my husband saw what I saw. In his calm, clinical manner he agreed: this was probably a seizure.

The next morning I stormed the pediatrician's office as politely as my panic would allow. The doctor sat with my son for some time and observed nothing remarkable. But he trusted enough in my convictions to refer us to a pediatric neurologist. A few weeks later, the specialist examined our son. He performed a full battery of neurologic tests disguised as play time for a full forty-five minutes before declaring Jonathan to be perfectly healthy. Reluctantly, and only at my insistence, he scheduled the child for a sleep electroencelphalogram (EEG). Only a few minutes into the test, my son had had so many seizures that the lab tech turned off the machine.

After reviewing the EEG results, the pediatric neurologist phoned, begging me to tell him, "How did you know?" He explained that children with this condition are rarely diagnosed with epilepsy until the second or third grade, when their inability to keep up in school raises developmental concerns. He could not believe that I had witnessed my son's seizures when he himself had been unable to detect any evidence of abnormality. Yet, in the time he spent interacting with my son, it is likely that the child experienced dozens of *absence* seizures. In response, I reminded him what many doctors forget: no one knows a child better than his mother.

Our story only begins to touch on some of the frustrations that accompany a diagnosis of epilepsy. It is an invisible disease with far-reaching and unpredictable effects. It can influence behavior, learning, and performance, but in ways that are not always apparent or well understood. Therefore, schools, employers, and society at large are oblivious to its hazards and fundamentally ignorant of how to accommodate those who are afflicted.

There is nothing my adult son wouldn't do today to give up the daily regimen of pills that has become his lifeline as well as his oppressor. I admire him for his strength and generosity in sharing his experiences, and for the hope and humor with which he approaches life. His memories, and the latent fears of someone living with a seizure disorder, are difficult to discuss. Epilepsy has many forms and manifestations, and all of them are isolating to children. Our hope is that something about our family's experience will resonate and help others to realize that they aren't alone.

Ellen Weiss Dodson

Coming to Terms

I do not remember being diagnosed with epilepsy. I was four years old. Given the frequency of doctor's visits, vaccines, nasty-tasting medicines, pokes and prods, it was just business as usual for me. But as I have come to understand, the world around me began to change. I was much more than ever under my mother's watchful eye. I required special handling at day care or when left with a babysitter. Even a simple playdate was not so simple anymore. There was a long list of dos and don'ts that followed me everywhere I went. And there was a new medication—a capsule filled with tiny sprinkles—the contents of which were scattered across my food twice a day.

It was the early 1990s. Many archaic social stigmas associated with epilepsy still lingered. One of my close relatives would only speak the name of the disease in a hushed whisper with her hand covering her mouth. Another harbored the long-held belief that epilepsy was 'possession by the devil' and thus remained in denial about my diagnosis, even to the point of refusing to serve up my medication while babysitting. As I reached young adulthood and pursued my own journey to understand my condition, I came to realize just how utterly misunderstood epilepsy is.

Epilepsy is not as rare as it may seem to the average person. Experts argue that there may be as many as 2.8 million (that's 8.4 out of every 1,000) people in the United States who suffer from some form of epilepsy. Compare this to other well know conditions that plague children and others, such as cerebral palsy (2.3 per 1,000), or juvenile diabetes (2.5 per 1,000). Epilepsy is more than three times more prevalent overall, yet it is overlooked by comparison. Research into causes and cures is grossly underfunded. Why? Because almost everyone with epilepsy experiences it in a different way. Some are debilitated by seizures while others lead lives that are relatively well-controlled by medication. Epilepsy has no consistent "face" or "brand," which makes it practically invisible to society at large. Indeed, until the age of twenty-one, I never knowingly met or saw another human being with epilepsy.

As I grew up, it didn't take long for the specter of epilepsy to cast its shadow on my life. It was difficult for me to cope. I could talk with my buddies about disdain for the math teacher or a crush on a pretty girl in class, but epilepsy was something I never shared. Carrying around this secret made me feel isolated and awkward. To make matters worse, I was pretty ignorant about it. All I really knew of the disease was what I saw in the mirror. I was epilepsy. I was broken, somehow. And I was alone.

There are no movie stars or public figures who rally the cause to fight epilepsy, to raise more research dollars, or to engender greater understanding for sufferers of this disease. The Ice Bucket Challenge brings awareness for Amyotropic Lateral Sclerosis (ALS)—also known as Lou Gehrig's disease. Michael J. Fox brings dignity and attention to Parkinson's disease. Like epilepsy, both ALS and Parkinson's are neurological diseases, but are degenerative and terminal—true plagues that deserve the support they get to find a cure. But have you ever seen the famous and fortunate walking the red carpet with purple lapel ribbons for epilepsy awareness? By contrast, epilepsy seems less dire. It is not a death sentence. Although the risk of seizures is commonly a lifetime affliction, the broad battalion of available neurological drugs helps the majority of epilepsy sufferers live well-controlled lives. Still, I am unashamed to admit the comfort it brought me when I discovered that hip-hop artist Lil Wayne, actor Danny Glover, and singer-songwriter Neil Young all suffer from seizure disorders. The late megastar Prince was also known to have suffered from epilepsy. These examples taught me that while epilepsy may be a speedbump on the road of life, I do not need to let it become a barrier.

Epilepsy is a broad term used when someone has experienced two or more seizures. Some people have seizures caused by tumors, fevers, injuries, vascular malformations, or other lesions. In my case, epilepsy is a *primary* diagnosis, meaning that I have seizures with no apparent underlying cause. Seizures may occur in just a portion or one hemisphere of the brain—these are called partial seizures. Mine are generalized seizures, meaning that electrical discharges occur in every part of my brain at once.

While doctors do not understand why seizures happen, they are highly recognizable on an EEG when they occur. For most people, normal brain activity acts much like the people running around Costco on a Sunday afternoon. Everyone has his or her own agenda, whether running to nab a gift-tin of cookies, a pup tent, a three-pack of drain cleaner, a big-screen TV, an enormous sack of rice, or a ridiculously large can of tuna. Now imagine that every person in the warehouse suddenly stops in place and jumps up and down three times in unison, repeating this synchronized three-beat pattern again and again for several seconds. This is what my brain is like when I am having a seizure. It is not a power failure; rather, it is an enormous power surge, causing my body to first stiffen and then shake. Afterward, I am left physically drained with no memory that this neurological "flash-mob" has occurred.

Neurologists—the doctors who treat epilepsy—focus their energy on preventing an epilepsy patient from having seizures. The anti-convulsive medicine I take provides a safety net, helping to calm the unpredictable irritability in my brain. Given too much medication, I am loopy, and rendered incapable of learning, working, driving, or operating machinery. Given too little, I am at risk for having a seizure without warning. Imagine that I could be using an electric saw, riding an escalator, carrying a tray of food to the table, or rocking a baby in my arms and suddenly lose control of my entire body.

Even fluctuations in the level of a therapeutic agent in the bloodstream can destabilize me. I take medication at 7:00 a.m. and 7:00 p.m. It sounds simple enough, but you'd be surprised how difficult it is to keep an appointment at a precise time every single day without exception. If I want to sleep late on vacation, I still have to wake up and take my meds. If I am at the movie theatre watching a new blockbuster, I still have to take my meds. Even if I am caught in a major traffic jam on the interstate, I still have to take my meds. And while the exact cause of seizures eludes us, there are known "triggers" that increase the risk of seizures. These include flashing or strobing lights, excessively loud noise, stress, exertion, lack of sleep, drugs, and alcohol. In my case, the combination of a late-night party, a hangover, a guilty conscience, and stress from a nagging mother is a perfect storm and almost always results in a seizure.

Writing this book is not going to give me a moment's rest from the burden of epilepsy that I have been carrying for the last twenty-five years. And thus far in my vast lifetime of experience, I doubt that I have uncovered or unlocked any secrets to making a child's diagnosis of epilepsy any less frightening or burdensome to them or their family. What I have discovered, however, is that society's tolerance and understanding of epilepsy and its effect on students and their families has progressed very little since man first walked on the moon. We need to talk more and to understand more—not just about the medical aspects of diagnosis and treatment. We need to understand how to best support patients and their families, so that a life lived with epilepsy can still mean a fruitful and productive life. Let's start that conversation.

● ● ● ● ●

http://www.epilepsy.com/learn/epilepsy-statistics (1/7/2016)
http://www.diabetes.org/diabetes-basics/statistics/ (1/8/2016)
http://cerebralpalsy.org/about-cerebral-palsy/prevalence-and-incidence/ (1/8/2016)

Flunking the Test

An EEG is a neurological test that reveals patterns of electrical activity in the brain. Because seizure activity is more likely to occur during "REM" sleep (REM stands for rapid eye movement, which happens when you are in a deep sleep), the EEG lab asked that I be restricted to less than four hours of sleep the night before the exam so that I would fall asleep quickly and sleep deeply during the exam. None of this can be explained to a four-year-old. Not the concept of diagnostic testing. Not the importance of staying forcibly awake well past your normal bedtime. Even during those childhood cartoon-loving years, there are only so many times you can watch a *Teenage Mutant Ninja Turtles* video into the night before you want to kill yourself.

Between my mother and father, mom lost the coin toss, which meant it was her job to keep me awake through the night. At first, it was fun having my favorite blanket spread on the living room floor while we sat, pic-nic-style, eating popcorn and watching movies. I was a big fan of Ted Turner's Earth-conscious superhero, singing at the top of my lungs, "Captain Planet! He's our hero! He takes pollution down to zero!" I even loved kicking up my heels with the dishes during *Beauty and the Beast's* "Be Our Guest" production number. By 11:00 p.m., our selection of videos and my mother's vast knowledge of Disney lyrics began to wear thin. I could not keep my eyes open.

Suddenly my mother rose. "Jonathan, let's put on your coat. We are going to the store!" she announced. Mom hoisted me into my car booster seat wrapped in my footed pajamas and cozy coat, accompanied by my trusty side-kick, a fluffy white, Dole-banana-toting, plush gorilla nicknamed Nana, (which is short for "Bananarilla").

One of the greatest inventions in American civili-zation is the twenty-four-hour supermarket. A veritable mecca for swing shift workers, delinquent teenagers, and working moms, we pressed the local Publix market into service as our all-night entertainment arcade. We began in the produce department. Mom found a banana that I could hold just like Nana's, cheering enthusiastically when I declared its color to be 'lellow.' There were apples, the many varieties of which I identified as red, yellow and green. We counted orange carrots tied in bunches to see which one had the most. We played "I Spy!" until I found the purple eggplant. We sought out all the items that were circles, including grapes, melons and oranges. With each success, my mother clapped her hands and squealed "Yay!" which elicited the most judgmental and hateful stares from nearby shoppers. After all, by this time it was well after midnight, long past the acceptable standard for dragging a pajama-clad toddler into the market.

As I lost interest in fruits and vegetables, my mother

made "zoom-zoom" sounds, pretending our shopping cart was an imaginary, souped-up race car. We sped to the can aisle, popping a wheelie along the way. I was oblivious to the vegetables in all the cans, but delighted to find all sorts of alphabet letters printed on them. Since the aisle was organized alphabetically, we called out the letters, navigating from artichokes to beets to corn and ending with yams and zucchini. On the kitchen supply aisle, my mother made a game out of picking up various sizes and shapes of aluminum roasting pans and asking, "Is this a hat?" We took turns trying on the ridiculous objects and giggling uncontrollably, inviting more scorn from the reluctant late-night shopper-zombies.

Next was the frozen food aisle. My mother picked me up out of the shopping cart and went to the first freezer case. She opened the door and pushed my face inside until I could feel the chill on my chubby cheeks. "Ooh! So cold," she squeaked in her playful mom voice. Then she hugged me tight, whispering into my ear, "*Sooo* warm!" She repeated this tango of cold and warm sensations at every door until we reached the end of the aisle.

On the soft drink aisle, I counted aloud proudly while mom placed one then two then three two-liter bottles in our cart, continuing to count until we reached ten. She let me demonstrate these skills a second time as we relocated them from the cart to the conveyor belt at checkout. Back in my car seat I fell asleep almost instantly, hardly waking as my mother carried me into the house and tucked me into my bed for four hours of sanctioned sleep time.

The next morning I was understandably cranky. Not only was I sleep-deprived, but I also sensed that things weren't as they should be. On this particular morning, I was allowed to take Nana in the car, and my mother didn't take the familiar turn to the day-care center where

I played happily with my friends each day. Instead, we got on the highway to make the trek to the children's hospital.

I didn't like that place from the moment we stepped inside. Seeking retreat, I pulled at my mother until she picked me up. We sat in a waiting room, uncertainty looming.

A nurse emerged in a white lab coat and attempted to lead me away. My mother asked to come into the procedure room, but the nurse refused her. She explained that I was required to sleep and that my mother would be a distraction. My mother thanked her politely, but insisted on coming anyway.

An EEG involves attaching more than twenty electrodes to different parts of the scalp in order to record brain activity. It is not invasive or painful, but it is awkward and uncomfortable to sit still while the electrodes are stuck to the head with paste. In one hospital, where I later had an EEG as an adolescent, they parted my hair and rubbed my bare scalp with sand paper in order to reduce resistance on the electrodes. This first time, it took more than an hour to place the electrodes. This four-year-old was having none of it. Every time the nurse attempted to touch my head or bring an electrode near me, I squirmed away, terrified.

My mother watched the nurse grow more and more impatient with my behavior. Finally, Mom said to the nurse, "If you want to get this done, just put an electrode on his stuffed gorilla."

The nurse looked at my mother and then at Nana and frowned. "I don't have time for this. We're just going to have to start an IV and put him to sleep."

"Over my dead body," my mother said, glaring in defiance. "Trust me," she said. "Just put one on the gorilla."

Begrudgingly, the nurse found some first-aid tape and attached one of the electrodes to my furry, stuffed companion, all the while mumbling under her breath in disgust. Then, my mother explained this bizarre scenario to me. She said that I was going to have a brain test and that Nana was going to have it first, just to show me that it didn't hurt. She allowed me to inspect the electrode and to see how it was stuck on Nana. She further explained that because Nana "was a baby" he only needed one wire, but that I was a big boy and would have a whole bunch. It wasn't going to hurt at all—it would probably tickle a bit—but I had to sit still so they didn't fall off.

My mother was right. The electrodes didn't hurt, but I felt very self-conscious and it itched to have them pasted all over my head. When it came time to sleep, there was no cot or bed in the tiny room. The nurse expected me to lie atop a butcher-paper-covered exam table and fall asleep. Again, my mother was incredulous. Without a word, she climbed up onto the small pediatric exam table herself. The nurse started to protest, but my mother put a hushing finger to her lips and stared her down. Mom stretched across the table the best she could with her legs hanging off. She held me close, spooning me while I, in turn, spooned Nana. In two minutes I was fast asleep in her arms.

Ten minutes later the nurse shut off the EEG machine. I had so many seizures in those first ten minutes that there was no need to continue for the full forty minutes in order to obtain a positive diagnosis of epilepsy.

It has been twenty-five years since that day. I confess that I can no longer distinguish between my own memories and the pictures that have been painted by hearing this story told again and again through the years. I still smile when I realize how ferocious my mother could be, advocating on my behalf in a health system that was often impersonal, fragmented, and clueless. And when I grow frustrated with my mother for the way her "love" sometimes feels oppressive or smothering, I remember her selfless and creative efforts to maintain my comfort and to shield me from what must have been her own unspeakable terror in the face of a frightening diagnosis.

Turn the Other Cheek

So now I am a spirited four-year old with a diagnosis of epilepsy.

My parents made up a busy, two-career power couple. They had no idea what this new reality would mean for our family. They did not know what steps to take to accommodate the uncertainty that is epilepsy's constant companion. There were so many concerns: Had my life's trajectory been forever altered? Would I require special care? Special schools? Would my mother be able to continue her work as a busy executive, with all the travel and long hours it entailed? And what about my new baby sister who just joined our family? The doctors warned there could be a hereditary component to my condition. Would my baby sister develop epilepsy too? How would my needs affect the life upon which she had barely embarked?

I was not aware that life as our family knew it had changed forever. I was too young to experience that surreal moment of shock that my mother describes, when everything stood very still and artificially tinted like in a cartoon. My parents felt completely blindsided. Epilepsy was an unwelcome and very demanding guest. This was something they knew nothing about, and they were powerless to fix it.

As for me, my diagnosis meant two immediate changes to my lifestyle. The first was the need to take an anti-convulsive medication. The doctor explained that although to date I had experienced only *absence* seizures (*absence* is pronounced with a French accent, as ab-SAHNS), the EEG patterns revealed that I was also likely to experience "tonic-clonic" seizures. *Absence* and tonic-clonic are the newer, more acceptable terms replacing the seizure labels *petit mal* and *grand mal* that were familiar to my grandparents' generation. Rather than using those archaic, ominous terms that, literally, mean "little bad" and "big bad," we now describe seizures by their clinical characteristics.

Absence seizures are brief disruptions to consciousness, lasting a moment or two with no aftereffect. You might not notice someone experiencing an *absence* seizure, or you might catch someone in an unresponsive stare that ends after a few seconds. A tonic-clonic seizure, by contrast, is a major event. During the tonic phase, the person loses consciousness and experiences a stiffening of their muscles, often falling down whether standing or sitting. During the clonic phase, the person's muscles contract in ways that appear as twitches, vibrations, or violent shakes. Commonly, the eyes will roll back in the head. It is not hard to understand why, for centuries, tonic-clonic seizures caused ignorant people to think sufferers of epilepsy were victims of witchcraft or possessed by the devil.

Because my particular type of epilepsy included both the *absence* episodes I was having regularly as well as tonic-clonic seizures, which I had not yet experienced, my doctor prescribed the medication Depakote, a substance that provided a broad-spectrum safety net to protect against the larger type seizures. At the time, Depakote was a newer drug, considered preferable to the longstanding Dilantin and Phenobarbitol, which cause inconvenient side effects, such as drowsiness, that can prove detrimental to the development of a school-age child.

I was fortunate that my medication could be taken in twelve-hour intervals, with breakfast and dinner. I never had to deal with taking pills at school. Also, Depakote came in a form designed for young children. It was dispensed as a big capsule filled with tiny medicinal sprinkles. My mother would open the capsule and sprinkle the medicine over a spoonful of applesauce or chocolate pudding and stick it in my mouth. As burdens go, this wasn't a tough one.

But remember I said there were *two* major changes to my lifestyle?

The thing about Depakote is that it is not well metabolized by children. This means that I had to take excess amounts of the drug just to get enough to stay in my bloodstream to fight the seizures. The doctor used my size and weight to estimate an initial dosage, then fine-tuned it to find my sweet spot, known as the "therapeutic range." If not enough Depakote was retained in my system I could have break-through seizures. Too much Depakote would put me at risk of liver damage. A Depakote regimen, therefore, required getting blood tests every month to measure liver function as well as medication levels in the bloodstream.

I had never had a blood test before. At first, I was just glad it wasn't another brain test. I sat quietly next to mother in the waiting room of that same children's hospital until a skinny guy came out and called my name. We followed Skinny Guy into another area where my mother sat in a stiff chair with me on her lap. Skinny Guy grabbed my arm and wrapped it way too tight with something sticky. Then he wiped my arm and made it feel cold and wet. Suddenly, he stuck something in my arm and I started to scream. I tried to get away from the pain, but found that my mother trapped my legs between hers. Skinny Guy was holding the arm with the pain, so with the other arm I reached around and dug my fingers as deep as I could into my mother's face.

I continued to scream and squirm while Skinny Guy pasted a Power Rangers band-aid across the bend in my arm. My mother pushed me off her lap and onto my feet. I looked back at her through my tears and saw where my claw marks were beginning to weep blood across her cheek. Although the pain in my arm was long gone, I continued to cry and twist at my shirt in frustration. I could not get my head around what I had just experienced. I was whimpering and limp, while my mother carried me back to the car while humming soothingly into my ear.

A few weeks later, I was happily riding in the car when I recognized the primary colored signage of that darned children's hospital. "No, no, no, no, no, no, no, NO, NO, NO, NOOO!" I started quietly and got louder and louder until my own voice was ringing painfully in my ears. The second my mother unclipped me from my car seat, I slithered away deep into the minivan, hoping to be beyond her reach. Somehow, my mother prevailed, carrying me away under her arm like a large, limp football.

This time the waiting room was filled with children. Remaining trepidatious, I watched them play with the generic collection of used toys, wondering if they were all about to meet a fate similar to mine. First a girl, and then a boy, disappeared behind the door and into the dreaded Chamber of Horrors. The girl emerged soon after and ran to her waiting mother; they left without drama. Then the boy emerged. There were no screams or whimpers, just a telltale band-aid on his arm suggesting that he had done battle with Skinny Guy. I collected myself, reasoning that perhaps the pain I recalled of the blood test had been a dream—a bad dream. Certainly my mother—my protector—would not allow that to happen to me again.

Skinny Guy appeared, reading my name from the clipboard he held in his hand. This time, my mother led me to him and returned to her seat. Shocked, I held my hands out for my mother and screamed. She smiled sweetly and blew me a kiss just as I disappeared into the Chamber of Horrors, led by the cold and unrelenting Skinny Guy.

It would be easier to describe what happened next behind the closed doors of the lab if you imagine my experience as a *Road Runner* cartoon. The coyote dropped down a chute, got hit over the head with a hammer, bounced from rock to rock, fell from a cliff, got hurled from a giant catapult, landed in the tree tops, fell to the ground, got smashed by a steamroller, yet at some unknown point along the way the intrepid little bird managed to extract a small vial of blood from his arm. Exhausted and reeling with hurt feelings, I returned to the waiting room whimpering and marked once again with a Power Rangers band-aid.

These monthly trips to the lab became such a horror in my life that I began to fear every instance of being in the car alone with my mother, certain that we were heading in that direction. Then one day, I was visited by an angel. She was, in fact, an old friend of my parents' whose husband had once been roommates with my dad. Her name was Bosch, and she worked as a nurse on the Navajo reservation in Shiprock, New Mexico. She specialized in helping diabetic patients comply with their insulin regimens. I asked her, "What can I do to keep my blood tests from hurting?"

Bosch gave my query some deep thought. "Well," she said, "your brain can't feel pain in two places at once. So why not try pinching your cheek?" I pinched my cheek then and there. It hurt, but it was a hurt I could manage. Alone in my room, I practiced pinching my cheek, making sure that the confidence it brought me the first time returned. Suddenly, I couldn't wait to try this at my next blood test!

Soon enough, the day arrived for my monthly trip to the children's hospital lab. I got in the car, buckled the straps around me on my booster seat, and grabbed my left cheek hard. I kept pinching it, continuing to assure myself that I could handle the scary needle if all I could feel was this grasp of my cheek. I pinched for the entire duration of the thirty-minute drive to the hospital. I pinched while we walked from the patient parking lot to the blood lab. I pinched while we sat in the waiting room anticipating the site of Skinny Guy. When he finally appeared and called my name, I turned to kiss my mother good-bye before heading bravely into the Chamber of Horrors. "Oh, Jonathan!" she cried out in a sinking tone. "Look what you've done to your face!"

My mother pulled a small compact mirror from her purse to show me. Across my cheek was an enormous bruise—a pink and purple "pinch hickey." She planted a kiss on it, but I remained focused on my mission. With complete confidence I marched up to Skinny Guy, clutching my cheek between my thumb and index finger. In a matter of minutes, I returned from the lab with my Power Rangers band-aid and a big smile across my face. "It worked!" I cried. "It worked! The blood test didn't hurt at all!"

Life is full of serendipitous moments. Honestly, I do

not know how I would have survived a childhood on Depakote had Nurse Bosch not visited on the day that she did. In all, I was on Depakote for seven years. That's well over eighty monthly trips to the lab to test my Depakote levels and liver function. I am no longer afraid of needles, but truth be told, I still reach up to my cheek each time I extend my arm for bloodwork.

Free Period

T here was only one time in my life when I
lived free of the baggage of epilepsy. When
first diagnosed with epilepsy, the doctors
called it "pediatric *absence*," offering me a
better than 50-percent chance that I would
outgrow my seizures. There is so little known
about the cause and course of epilepsy, but
oftentimes the far side of puberty can result in
stabilization of the erratic brain activity associated with childhood seizure disorders.

By the age of eleven, my family had moved
from Atlanta to the Boston area. I had been
on Depakote for most of my young life. And
my voice was slowly descending into a
mellow baritone. We were referred to a
well-known specialist at a local children's hospital to continue my epilepsy
care. At my first appointment, I was dis-
patched to the EEG lab before the doctor
would even see me. Conducted without
advanced notice and therefore without sleep

deprivation, I survived the stimulation of all the triggers without manifesting a seizure.

The new doctor asked when I had last experienced a seizure. It had been two years. My last seizure had been triggered during a routine, sleep-deprived EEG during which I was subjected to strobe lights and hyperventilation. In the world of pediatric neurology, puberty plus two years seizure-free is a watershed moment. It is an indication that the patient may have outgrown his childhood epilepsy.

The doctor also made note of the fact that I had been on a consistently high dose of Depakote for many years. After about two years with the children's sprinkle capsules, I learned to swallow a big pill whole with water. My dosage was now higher than what was typically prescribed for adults. "Let's start weaning you down off the Depakote," the doctor said. "At this age," he explained, "your body will metabolize the drug more efficiently, which probably means you will be able to achieve therapeutic levels on a lower dose."

People with epilepsy are exquisitely sensitive to changes in drug levels, so any change in drug or dosage must be managed in a slow, incremental manner. The doctor made a schedule where I would decrease the amount of Depakote I took by a specific amount every two weeks. He said to my mom, "Call me when he has a break-through seizure and we'll go from there."

We went home and taped my eighteen-week dose-reduction schedule to the refrigerator. I continued to take my medicine at my usual twelve-hour intervals, but at each two-week milestone, either my morning or evening dose would be decreased by a small amount. The pharmacist gave us pills in various doses that could be cut up and combined to make the appropriate dose for each stage in the schedule. I continued my normal routine of school, homework and my new love—hockey. Soon, winter hockey ended and Little League season began. Though right-handed at hockey, I played first base left-handed and was a switch hitter. Our team made the playoffs and won the league championship.

When we began the weaning schedule, the plan was to discover and adjust to a new, lower therapeutic dose of Depakote. But the seizures never came. I kept going until one day my evening dose was at zero and my morning pill was down to the smallest increment. My mother watched me closely for those last two weeks, picking me up at school and attending every baseball game. We came to the end of the doctor's hand-scribbled schedule.

My mother called the doctor and asked him what to do next.

"You're done!" he said.

"Just like that?" my mother asked. "Don't you want to examine him or do an EEG? Just to make sure he's OK?"

"Go away and count your blessings," he said.

"No meds at all? Do you want to see him in a year?" she asked, still not believing that there wasn't more to it all.

"Ma'am," he said impatiently, "I deal with a lot of very sick children. Your son hasn't had a seizure in over two years. What more do you want from me? If he has a seizure, then call me." He hung up the phone.

After school, my mother sat me down to share the news. I was finished with the pills and the blood tests. I felt like Pinocchio on the day he awakens to discover he is a real boy. I wanted to jump and run and fly—anything to feel alive and untethered.

"Can we celebrate?" I asked.

Together we planned a family fun night. We included my close friend, Ryan, whose mother let him out late with us on a school night. We went to an authentic Irish-style pub for dinner and then out to Jillian's, a legendary Boston fun factory next to Fenway Park. Jillian's has pool tables, bowling alleys, huge video monitors everywhere, and a video arcade. It was a collection of nearly every epilepsy hazard under one roof: loud music, clanging sounds, and flashing lights, all cranked up to eleven. My parents sat apprehensively and sipped drinks while I had the time of my life.

The next morning I woke up and instinctively reached for my medicine before grabbing breakfast. Taking pills had become so much a part of who I was, I felt almost naughty bypassing them. It was like going to school commando!

Within a few weeks I stopped reaching for the pill bottle. In a couple months I was at summer hockey camp with no restrictions on my activities. I swam, I dived, I climbed. I participated in everything. I could go to the house of a new friend without my mother's having to run through the litany of restrictions and seizure precautions. Finally, I could see epilepsy in my rear view mirror!

Here We Go Again

When you're a teenager, every year is a milestone. For each year older, the world opens its doors to more and more opportunities for young adults. At sixteen, I was feeling very grown up. I hit an unexpected and greatly welcome growth spurt, started to imagine life beyond high school, and enjoyed the attention of some very pretty girls. I was also looking forward to taking the road test for my driver's license.

I spent much of the summer before tenth grade in hockey camps, clinics, and leagues working to hone my puck-handling skills and build speed on the ice. I went to the gym every other day to lift weights, trying to bulk up my skin-and-bones one hundred-forty-pound frame. One hockey program was especially intense in its cross-training skills. We had overland relays, endurance competitions, military-style obstacle courses, and diving treasure hunts on the bottom of a lake.

It was now five years since my last dose of anti-convulsive medicine. Five years since my last blood test. In all honesty, I had blocked all memories of those days. I no longer saw myself as a kid with a disease or disability, although I was still very much an underdog athletically. I was a small kid trying to become big enough and fast enough to play high school hockey.

Youth hockey in New England is legendary. People take this stuff very seriously. Parents get very involved in the action. Some years back, in one infamous case, a parent of a player on one team assaulted a parent from another team, causing his death. Since then, players and parents alike must sign code of conduct agreements as a condition of participation. Parents are warned not to cheer exclusively for their own child or team; they must cheer equally for the accomplishments of their opponents. These legal formalities do not temper the intensity of youth hockey games. Even off-season games, like the fall leagues of early September, are well attended by boisterous logo-clad families and friends.

On opening day that fall, the rink was filled with familiar faces. We emerged from the stinky locker room and into the refrigerated air of the rink. In the stands I recognized the parents of my friends wrapped in fleece blankets, cute girls from school averting eye contact with practiced indifference, and my sister with her "younger-siblings club"—rink rats that ran up and down the bleachers and pressed their runny noses against the glass. We took our warm-up laps to the cheers of the home crowd, then stood cradling our helmets in our arms while a recording of the national anthem played over the scratchy PA system.

I skated out with my friends to center ice for the face-off, standing at center position with my stick poised.

The referee dropped the puck and I swatted at it, hoping it would make its way to a friendly stick. We played hard for thirty seconds—like bumpers on a pinball machine we sent the puck around and around the rink—and then dumped the rubber disk down the ice, retreating to the bench in a carefully choreographed switch to the second line. The door of the box slammed shut.

That's the last thing I remember.

● ● ● ● ●

There were voices all around me. They faded in and out. As much as I tried, I could not keep them there with me. I heard quiet voices. I heard distant voices squawking on a radio. I could not move.

" … to the hospital," I heard someone say. It was not a voice I recognized.

The haze came in and out in waves. I told myself to focus. My eyes were closed. I tried to open them, but could only hold them for a second. In my head I reviewed the faces I glimpsed under fluttering eyelids. Strangers, all. Where was I? Who were these men who were whispering? I only understood some of the words they were saying.

"…ictal," I heard. More squawking on that radio. Still can't move.

I attempted a mental inventory of my faculties. The smell of damp mold filled my nostrils! I was playing hockey. I tried to squeeze my hands, but I could not seem to find a grip. I tried to lift my legs but they did not move. Nothing felt right. My mind flashed to the image of a wall plaque at one of the nearby rinks. It was a cautionary tale and tribute to a local kid—one of the many young hockey players whose life had been forever altered by spinal injury. I panicked, wondering if that was what had happened to me. There was a tightness around my chest. I was uncomfortable and something was pinching my back. I tried again to lift my leg, but it was stuck in place.

"Jawn!" I heard someone say with a textbook Boston accent.

"Dammit," I yelled inside my head. "My name is not John. It's Jonathan!"

"Jon. A. Than," I tried to push the syllables out of my mouth. My mouth felt clumsy, my tongue seemingly twice its normal size. I blinked my eyes open and shut.

"Here he is," a warm voice said, sounding very much like my dad.

"Am … I … *paralyzed*?" I asked, almost afraid to verbalize a hockey player's greatest fear. There was a chuckle from beside me, then another near my feet. Who were these guys? Not my friends. Not my coach.

"Jonathan," the voice that sounded like my dad said. "You had a seizure, buddy. Everything is OK, but we have to take you to the hospital now."

"I'm not paralyzed?" I asked again, needing more confirmation. "Why can't I move?" Boy, was I tired. I kept my eyes closed.

The chuckler beside me was first to answer. "You are strapped to a gurney and you have all your hockey gear on. But we cut your laces and removed your skates. Just move your toes."

I wiggled my toes and then someone ran his finger up the bottom of my foot, causing me to flinch involuntarily. At this, I gulped in a deep breath. My worst fear was over.

Somewhere over my head I heard my mother. She spoke soothing mom things to me but her voice was all choked up. Was she crying? I tried to open my eyes again but only managed to squint. There were gauges and displays and medical equipment all around me. Two guys in uniform were busy taking readings and vital signs. There was a large plastic contraption embedded in my left arm; the arm was taped to a board. I could see the IV line pushing fluids into me. Someone told my dad that he could stay in the ambulance with me; my mother and sister would follow in the car. Doors slammed and we started to move, slowly at first and then faster and faster as the siren whined overhead.

During the ride my father caught me up on what had occurred. As soon as I completed my shift on the ice, I slid onto the bench with the other players. After a few seconds, I fell over onto the player next to me. My team-mate told me later that he thought I was joking around and was pushing me to sit up. When convulsions started, my coach stopped the game and sent all the players onto the ice to clear the box. They moved the wooden bench out of the way so I wouldn't hit my head. Someone called 911 and the fire rescue squad arrived almost immediately from up the street. I was unconscious following the sei-zure—known as a "post-ictal state"—for twelve minutes. During this period of non-responsiveness, I was loaded on a stretcher, carted off the ice, and placed in the ambu-lance. They cut holes in my socks to place heart monitors and started an IV.

"Well," I told my dad, looking at the plastic gadget protruding from my arm, "at least I didn't have to pinch my cheek!"

Everything at the children's hospital should have gone smoothly. I already had a record there where I had been seen years earlier for epilepsy, before being weaned off of medication. Everything about my incident was consistent with a rather large tonic-clonic seizure. But as it turns out, neither of my parents had witnessed the seizure, only the mayhem that followed. And since I had never had a tonic-clonic seizure before, they were a little freaked out by the prolonged unconsciousness that typically follows that type of seizure.

By the time I arrived at the emergency room, about twenty-five minutes had elapsed since the seizure. As is the case with epilepsy, I was tired but absolutely fine in a clinical sense. My mother explained my history of childhood seizures and that I had records here, in this very hospital. But to the staff physicians, I was only a teenager who blacked out playing hockey. Based on their expert medical opinions, they needed to run blood gases and work me up for a cardiac event.

My mother and father tried to intervene, insisting that this wasn't necessary. "He did not faint," they said. "This is a kid with a history of seizures who very likely just had his first tonic-clonic. He doesn't need blood gases, he needs an EEG!" The doctor refused, explaining that it was against policy to perform an EEG on an outpatient.

"So, admit him," my mother insisted. "He has been seizure-free for years, but there was always a known probability the seizures could return. Today is that day!"

"There is nothing wrong with him to justify admission," the doctor explained. "But we do need to rule out any cardiac problems as a reason he might have fainted. We will need to check his blood gases."

Exasperated at their inability to focus the doctors on the real culprit, my parents gave way to allow them to draw blood. Because I had that giant IV contraption placed in my arm already, they extracted blood by reversing the pressure in the tubing. My whole family watched as blood traveled out of my arm and around the cloverleaf curves of the plastic gadget, through another tube, and spilled out into the necessary vials. My sister, who was twelve, took one look, turned white as a ghost, and hit the floor.

The ER nurse called for another gurney and placed my sister's limp little body on it. They brought in another set of monitors and hooked her up so that her heart rate and mine pinged in syncopated rhythms from opposite sides of the exam room. At this point, I was no longer of any concern to anyone in the emergency room. A medical team surrounded my sister, who, normally would have been chatting away like any normal tween. Instead, she was horrified and tongue-tied, and possibly in shock. Her blood pressure was barely ninety over sixty and her heart rate was only forty-one beats per minute. We all listened while the medical team discussed transferring her to the ICU.

My father tightened his lips and shook his head. My mother looked like she was going to explode, right there, all over the emergency room. My sister and I were both laid out on beds and attached to monitors. I started to laugh. I had just had the mother of all seizures and the hospital refused to do an epilepsy work up. In the meantime, my sister, who was a prize-winning juvenile figure skater—athletic teen girls are known to have low blood pressure—fainted at the sight of blood and had the whole staff ready to perform open-heart surgery.

My mother pointed her finger at every medical person in the room. "No one goes anywhere until I get back!" she ordered.

She disappeared and returned a few minutes later, her arms filled with orange packages of Reese's Peanut Butter Cups. She unwrapped a piece of candy and stuck it, whole, into my sister's mouth. "Swallow that," she commanded. My sister happily complied.

"Again," my mother pushed a second one into her

mouth. She slowly increased her tempo and volume, trying to get my sister to fight back. "Another!"

Suddenly struck by the ridiculousness of it all, my mother couldn't help laughing, which started my sister laughing too. The color came back into her cheeks and she felt fine, but her heartrate remained low, despite my mother's best efforts to ruffle her feathers. The ranking physician insisted she was bound for the ICU.

Now, my father is the calmest and most patient man I know. But as a doctor who does not suffer fools, he had had enough. He stepped out of the room and returned twenty minutes later with a fistful of rolled up paperwork. "We are going home," he announced sternly. "Now!"

On the long ride home my father explained that there was nothing the medical team could or would do for me despite the fact that I had clearly experienced a seizure and needed to resume treatment for epilepsy. As for my sister, they insisted she be admitted to the ICU—which would have begun with their trying to start an IV on her, too. Instead of arguing, dad signed the legal forms required to facilitate her release "against medical advice." We laughed at the irony all the way home.

Although the experience at the hospital unfolded like a whacky sitcom, once the shock wore off, a new reality set in—my reality. Lying in my own room later and sleeping it off I realized that my life had just taken a critical turn. It had been years. I had forgotten, or maybe blocked, the memories of a childhood with epilepsy. It all came flooding back to me now: the disruptive blood tests, the necessary precautionary disclosures to friends, teachers and coaches, the yearly EEGs, and the rhythm of the pills. Oh, the pills! Objects so small, yet they disempowered me. They were not only a constant reminder of my affliction. Each pill I swallowed was an act of submission that reinforced epilepsy's complete control over my life.

This sort of news is very different to receive at sixteen than at four. I had been publicly outed by my seizure during the spectacle of a packed ice rink. Word spread quickly through the high school grapevine. By the time I returned from the hospital I had more than a hundred text messages—some stupid, some mocking, and many showing real concern. How would I explain this? I had never confronted the stigma of epilepsy, and yet my first instinct was that this was something I wanted to hide, to deny. How could I quiet the churning rumor mill? Could I lie to people about what they had clearly witnessed? And was this just a freak occurrence, or would I now start having random drop seizures as often as I once had *absence* seizures? What did this all mean for my life going forward?

I would like to say I was brave as my new reality unfolded. In truth, I felt sorry for myself. I wondered why this was happening to *me*. Why were seizures coming back after all these years? And now I had to contend with a very different sort of seizure than before. Why was I the one in my family who had to suffer with this? Was there something I did that caused seizures to reawaken in me. What if people who had been my friends for years would suddenly treat me differently? Would I be able to play the hockey I loved? And what about all my other plans for the future?

The answers to these questions were slow to unfold. During that time I was very isolated with my fears. After all, who could understand what I was going through? The one bright spot of good news is that my new doctor was recommending a new drug—Lamictal—that did not require liver function tests. So while I would again be a slave to twice daily medications, the monthly blood tests would remain in the past. It was a small victory, but this one piece of good news gave me hope. And the more I considered what I had been through, it galvanized me to realize that I was handling it. I handled it before and I could certainly do it again.

Six months to the day after the hockey incident, having satisfied the restrictions of state law regarding seizures, I passed the road test and was issued a Massachusetts driver's license.

Normal

My high school was one of the most fiercely competitive public schools in the Northeast. Its graduates were the favorites of Ivy League Admissions counselors. One graduate after another attained high SAT scores, better than a 4.0 grade-point average, and state recognition in orchestra, debate, or science Olympiad. Although they came in all shapes, sizes, and ethnicities, my fellow students were oddly indistinguishable from one another on paper—such were the heights of their academic achievements. They knew it was not enough to simply deliver the grade. One had to stand out from the crowd—this tough crowd—to capture the prize of Ivy League admission. It was entertaining to watch the ways these students tried to outdo each other in the college sweepstakes.

Everyone around me was trying to break academic records in order to stand out. As for me, I was just trying to be normal. 'Normal' was my White Whale.

My particular brand of epilepsy manifests as abnormal electrical activity in all parts of my brain. On medication, I maintain a narrow window between a slightly unstable electrically charged irritability and a full-on seizure state. Even though I am considered well controlled on medication, I always have sub-clinical abnormal brain activity. Always. Normal? Never!

In social situations, I probably seem perfectly normal to most people, but I have become aware to the point of self-consciousness of my own physical and cognitive limits. For example, I am not great multi-tasker. I am more comfortable when I can focus linearly on one topic or task at a time. For this reason, I do far better in school taking an essay exam, which allows me to explain what I know, than with a multiple choice exam, where I need to sort through three or four ideas at once. And I can think far more clearly when not racing against a ticking time clock. Timed tasks are a severe barrier for me. The fear of running out of time affects me physiologically, causing me to hyperventilate which, in turn, increases the frequency of abnormal "spikes" of electrical activity in my brain.

In retrospect, an academic pressure-cooker high school was the wrong fit for someone who struggles to be normal. In my school environment, I felt at risk for public humiliation every day—and every minute of every day. Seizures occur most often under stress conditions. The demand to perform multiple complex tasks causes stress. Class participation causes stress. Timed tasks cause stress. Disappointment in my own performance causes stress. And the stress of knowing that a seizure is imminent causes stress. Because if there is one thing that every kid with epilepsy knows, it's that this disease looms large. There is always a seizure lurking. It is not a matter of *if* but *when*. There is no hiding from it, or cheating on lifestyle norms, or taking a vacation from the medications. It's a burden that gets heavier and heavier as time goes on.

I found living with the uncertainty of epilepsy to be exhausting. It is like dueling with an invisible opponent. I cannot see it, and yet it keeps sucker-punching me. Such was the case when the whole town witnessed the return of my seizures. Nothing cuts a cool dude down to size quicker than becoming a public spectacle. Here I was, trying to disappear into the crowd and instead I was the trending topic of the week! It did not help matters when the emergency respondents pointed out that my seizure was now on record, prohibiting me by state law from driving for a full six months. Not only was I miserable that my seizures had returned but I was also forced to endure the mortal shame of being driven to hockey practice by my mother while all my friends were driving themselves.

Years later, when I studied sociology in college, the 'normal' that I used to benchmark my life took on new meaning for me. I learned that we superimpose a lot of limits and barriers across society, creating artificial or "socially constructed" ideas of what normal is. We have a tendency to consider things that are in the majority or most familiar as normal, and then cast labels of abnormal on everything else.

After all, aren't we raised to appreciate "sameness" as a virtue? From the earliest age, we are taught to scorn the outlier. We sing along with Big Bird that "One of these things is not like the other. One of these things just doesn't belong." We heed our primal call to cling to "our own kind," arranging ourselves instinctively into tribe-like cliques and gangs. During my elementary years, I had a lot of Catholic friends who attended CCD training, which culminated with their First Holy Communion in the spring. They emerged with shiny gold crosses around their necks signifying their faith, completing their religious right of passage. In a different part of town, I attended Hebrew School and stood publicly at the age of thirteen to declare my manhood and my Jewish faith. I begged my mother for a gold "chai" pendant so that I, too, could proudly brandish the symbol of my "tribe." It made me feel normal and included.

Through my education I learned to appreciate how superficial and ultimately dangerous imposing labels on people can be. While we identify with those who have like characteristics and values in order to feel comfortable or included, aren't we also drawing a line between us and others, thereby excluding them from our company? We are a world divided by Coke and Pepsi, by Yankees and Red Sox, by Democrats and Republicans. People speak commonly of "we" and "they." Bias is so ingrained in our culture that when we happen to fall within the majority we barely see the burden that that framework places on others. I still remember the sting I felt when a teacher pointed out how common it is to call to George Clooney an "actor" while referring to Denzel Washington as a "black actor." Bias—in the forms of racism, sexism, bigotry and privilege—is everywhere in our culture and our institutions. We can't help judging the people around us, using our own privilege as a yardstick.

These educational revelations only made me more self-conscious about the invisible quirks of epilepsy and how they made me different. I sought to be normal for its anonymity and the sense of belonging. It was ironic to me that kids in my high school aspired to become overachievers—outliers to be singled out and thrust into the spotlight. I sought the comforting shadows of lower expectations. As I got older and found schoolwork even more challenging, I refused to seek the accommodations and special assistance that are available to students with disabilities, such as increased time allowances for tests. To me, being treated different reinforced the fact that I was different. I preferred taking the same classes under the same terms as everyone else, even though it often reflected unfavorably in my grades. Being an average student in an exceptional high school was a big victory for me. I wasn't proud of my grades, exactly, but they got me where I needed to go.

College and Self~Knowledge

As far back as I can remember I dreamed of attending the University of Oregon, my father's alma mater. My father is a great man in so many ways: professor, scholar, surgeon, athlete, and giant. I mean the latter in its most literal sense. In his prime, he stood six-foot-four. By the time I reached fifteen years old, it was clear by my five foot six stature—an unappreciated "gift" from a childhood spent taking Depakote—that I would never hit the six-foot mark. Well, if I couldn't reach my father's height, I reasoned, at least I could try to walk in his shoes. His green-and-yellow laced, fighting-Duck adorned, Nike-stamped, "JUST-DO-IT" University of Oregon shoes.

During my junior year in high school, Dad took me on a college tour across his home state of Oregon where we looked at a variety of viable college choices. My mother and my school counselor—ever practical—were both pushing for me to attend one of the smaller schools where I would not get lost in the crowd and could get individualized attention appropriate to my needs. Oregon has several smaller colleges that interested me. I had good interviews, exciting the admissions counselors with the possibility of attracting someone from such an exotic, faraway locale as Boston.

The last stop on the tour was the University of Oregon campus in Eugene. Normally a stoic man, it was obvious by the look in his eyes that Dad was greatly moved to be escorting his only son around his former stomping grounds. He showed me the austere hole-in-the-wall where he lived on campus. I wondered what secrets of his heyday hijinks lingered in those hallowed halls. We walked through buildings where he had labored through English and chemistry classes, stealing into an empty lecture hall to sit quietly together—one of us facing his future while the other reflected upon his past. My father shares little about himself with others, but while showing me his college he came as close as ever to baring his soul. I never really understood raging loyalty to one's alma mater, but there my father was, basking in the remembered glory of his Wonder Years. It was clear this university, with its angry Disney mascot and unlikely color combination, runs through his veins and vigorously pumps his heart. It brought my image of the man into sharper focus. I felt the connection from father to son, and so I made a connection to this university. What was once my childhood dream stood before me now as an imperative, a birthright. I was determined to make this my school, too.

I was never afraid of venturing three-thousand miles away for college. Honestly, it baffled me just how many of my friends wanted to go to school within a stone's throw of home. I could not imagine being close enough to come home on weekends, even if it meant foregoing the raptures of my mother's home cooking and clean, freshly folded laundry. I love my mother's chimichurri steak, but I wanted more than anything to live life on my own. I wanted to prove that I could manage my life, which, of course, meant owning my epilepsy.

But taking the reins was trickier than I realized.

When you grow up with a disability, whether physical or medical, it is always the elephant in the room. My parents were sensitive enough not to dwell on it, but I could always sense my mother's discerning and protective eye. She found a way to ensure that my activities avoided the standard epilepsy don'ts: climbing, swimming underwater while holding my breath, and using powered machinery. She discouraged me from attending concerts, parties, or dances where there might be a disco ball or strobing lights. She scrutinized my itinerary before I drove off, mentally screening for potential epilepsy hazards. If I didn't return home on the exact minute of my curfew, she would begin calling my cell phone non-stop, one call after another, until I answered and assured her I was safe. When we rode in the car together, she would casually point at something off the road when an ambulance came streaming by, just to ensure that I did not stare into its flashing red lights. Clearly, my health and safety weighed heavily upon her always.

It took some years before I appreciated the caring more than I resented the smothering.

My mother was obsessed with my pills. (Truth be told, she still is.) When living with epilepsy, pills are as important as the air you breathe. Stability relies on maintaining a perfect rhythm in your medication consumption. My mother lived from dose to dose, frequently posing in the kitchen with my bottle of pills outstretched just as I careened down the stairs to grab them. Sometimes, when I had an important exam, she would text me in school to double-check that I had taken my morning meds. If I went straight to baseball practice or someone's house after school, my mother would track me down to make sure that I had a stash of extra pills along to swallow at dinnertime.

But my mother wasn't my only oppressor. My hockey coach treated me as if I had a brain injury or was some delicate creature who might crumble upon contact. He seldom let me play. Some of my teachers resented the difficulties I had in class and on exams, perceiving me as sloppy or lazy rather than struggling. As a medical diagnosis, my counselors equated having epilepsy with conditions like diabetes or irritable bowel syndrome. They felt that it was simply not a relevant matter. They had no appreciation or compassion for the cognitive and performance difficulties I faced on a daily basis. I was caught between being too able, they felt, for special assistance and yet too impaired to function at the high levels that were expected of me.

In retrospect, there was a clear demonstrated relationship between my ability to perform in class and my epilepsy. In fact, during my years off medication, I peaked academically, doing well in advanced-level classes. A sharp drop-off at the end of ninth grade, during which time I became easily distracted and less detail-oriented in my work, was probably an advanced sign that the seizures were about to return. I do not have attention deficit disorder (ADD), but prolonged concentration became tough for me. Nerves and stress cause an increase in my heart and breath rates, sometimes leading me to borderline hyperventilation before an important exam, such as a final or the all-important SAT. I have seen what these stressors do to my EEGs. Although my medications provide a safety net that protects me from the three-spiked formations that define a seizure, (remember the Costco jumpers?) heavy breathing and stress often bring me to a near-seizure level, manifesting on an EEG as one- and two-spiked irregular formations. As a result, I can master a topic well and yet fail to be able to recall my knowledge during an exam.

Academic performance wasn't the only thought that weighed on my mind as college approached. Epilepsy had been a bleak cloud overhead all through high school, since being outed by my public and widely gossiped-about hockey seizure. While the self-knowledge, the fear, the constant restriction, and the never-ending schedule of pills is socially isolating enough, I was also weary of peer ignorance and chin-wag. I was ready for a change. College was an opportunity to reinvent myself and to experience campus life as a normal kid. Distance and independence, I felt, were the keys to my happiness. So when the University of Oregon invited me to join their freshman class in Eugene, I was elated. I could hardly wait to make friends with strangers and, yes, to party hearty.

And I did. I look back at my freshman year in college and cringe at my unbridled behavior. To be honest, I was irresponsible and wild, believing that I could do it all and have it all. My grades, which are sadly and indelibly stamped on my permanent record, are a testament to my lack of self-control. A large campus always has distractions. If one of my buddies had to write a paper or study for an exam, I could always find someone else who was taking a night off with a six-pack of Pabst Blue Ribbon.

I tried my best to push my epilepsy deep to the back of my mind. Far away from home, there was no one who knew my secret identity as the kid with epilepsy. I was confident that my seizures would remain well controlled as long as I never missed a pill. I took them surreptitiously, while my roommate slept late in the mornings. Then at dinnertime someone would invariably ask what I was popping. "Vitamins," I would lie. "Don't worry about it."

My parents lectured me non-stop about limiting alcohol consumption—not just because of the inherent risks of abuse, but also because of alcohol's effect on the brain. Studies show that drinking can reduce the half-life of some epilepsy medications. Before leaving for college, I asked my neurologist about drinking and she encouraged me to enjoy college life. "Having a beer isn't going to kill you," she said. I interpreted this as an unrestricted green light. I told myself, "Take your medicine and you can get drunk. Just make sure you remember to take it again in the morning!" I got through the first month without a seizure. Then another. I made it home for the holidays and was still seizure-free. Each milestone gave me more confidence, making me cocky. I convinced myself I had tamed the beast!

Memorial Day weekend arrived and spring finals were in sight. I had only one class on Friday, at 8:00 a.m., and then watched as the campus emptied out for the long weekend. Swarms of people flocked to Lake Shasta to enjoy an annual U of O tradition of raging on rented houseboats. I hadn't managed my money well enough to pull together the funds to go. Instead, I joined a bunch of buddies in a good old-fashioned, college-style party weekend. We were all underage, but it was easy to find friends who were older and willing to act as procurers of beer.

By Monday morning I was thoroughly trashed. I spent the day trying to recover from the mother of all hangovers. My head was pounding against my skull and my hands were shaking. I was too sick to sleep. I worried whether I'd be fit for the hockey scrimmage I committed to that night with the members of the U of O club team.

I really needed to get some food in me, but my stomach wasn't having any of it.

Somehow I managed to get myself to the rink. The acrid smell of the locker room was unbearable; I turned to the wall to hide the fact that I was gagging uncontrollably. I put my equipment on in the wrong order and then laced up my skates on the wrong feet. One of my teammates noticed that I was struggling to tape my stick and started laughing in my face. "I remember freshman year," he teased.

It was such a relief to hit the ice. The frigid air in the rink always has magical, resuscitative powers for me. I began to feel human again. That is, until my deluded world came crashing down.

A Cold One

" Jonathan?"

My head was pounding. I couldn't open my eyes, but I could hear voices all around me.

"Hey, Jon? Jon!"

"Is he OK?"

"I've never seen anything like *that* before."

"Did anyone see what happened?"

My arms and legs felt like anchors. I was exhausted—completely drained of every ounce of strength and will. I could not move. I tried, but I just could not open my eyes. In my head, I was trying to form the words, anything to let them know that I was still inside. Deep within this motionless body, I was here.

They were friendly voices. Familiar voices I could not identify. I could not reach out to the voices. The will to retreat into my inner cocoon was just too great. I did not have the strength. I needed to shut down and recharge my batteries.

"Who's got a cell phone? Somebody call 911! Quick!"

"Jonathan! Jon, buddy, everything is going to be all right."

"I think he had a seizure! My cousin has epilepsy, and that was definitely a seizure."

"That was so scary. Did you see what happened? He just got stiff and fell over on the ice."

"What do we do? Check whether he swallowed his tongue? Don't people do that?

Suddenly I was very cold. I could not remember being this cold before. I wanted to ask someone why it was so cold, but I still could not form any words. I was so tired; I wondered why. Had I just sprinted a marathon? No, I don't run. And I would be hot instead of cold. Such cold. Please make it stop.

"Hold on, buddy. We've got you." I knew the voice and could imagine the face that went with it, but could not quite put a name to it. It wasn't my mother or my father. Shouldn't they be here? Why aren't they here?

The excited chatter of familiar voices stopped. A different voice, one with authority, erased all the others.

"What happened? What is his name?"

"Jonathan!" I remembered, inside my head. My name is Jonathan. I am a college student and … a hockey player. I was playing hockey. My buddies are here. It was my shift and I went for the puck and … oh, shit! Not now! Not here! At the realization of what occurred, my heart sank.

"Son," the new voice said. I could feel him peel open my eyelid and scan my eye with an annoying light. "Can you hear me? You are OK. You might have had a seizure. Can you tell me your name? Has this happened before?"

I repeated my name, this time aloud. "Jonathan," I tried to say, but my ears told me that all I had managed was "Nannanon."

From inside my head I reached out to my body. I tried

to squeeze my hands, but I could not find a grip. I tried to wiggle my toes, but they did not move. My tongue! Oh, how my tongue was throbbing. During the seizure I had bitten it hard. I tasted the metallic taste of fresh blood. I wiggled it in my mouth to make sure it was all still there.

The unfamiliar voice was still speaking at me. Through the fog I heard "name" and "seizure."

"Jon-a-than," I tried again, this time articulating my name as best I could with my aching tongue. I pushed passed the need to recoil, to retreat back to the cocoon of numbness and sleep it off. For some reason it felt very important to communicate that I was alive and competent and in the moment. I could feel the stranger invading my space, touching me, poking at me. It was then that I realized I was in full hockey gear, the massive shoulder pads pressing into my back, my feet still bound snugly into my skates. I began to hear the clicking and clacking of an ambulance stretcher. I had been through this drill before.

Now, the fear set in, overtaking my very real need to sleep. Hospitals. IV tubes. Arguing with doctors that this was not a fainting spell. I do not require blood gases, or observation, or a thousand other diagnostic tests. "Epilepsy," I finally said out loud, not realizing that this was as much a confession to myself as it was an affirmation to the ambulance guy. And then with as much cool as I could muster, I added, "No big deal."

● ● ● ● ●

The post-ictal phase that follows a tonic-clonic seizure slowly subsided, and I regained my sense of time and place. I opened my eyes to see my closest buddies huddled on the ice around me: my brothers on blades. There

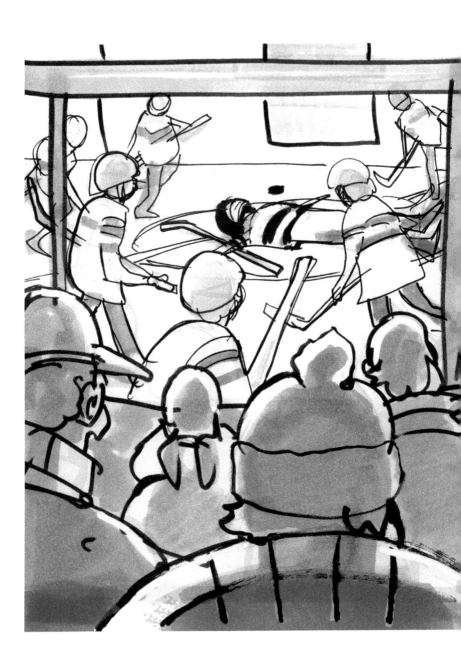

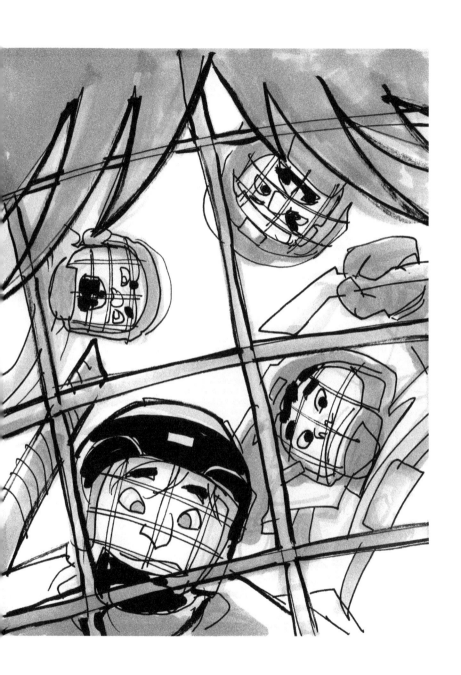

A COLD ONE

was no judgment or disgust at what they had witnessed, just looks of sincere concern. It was a moment that should have reassured me, but instead I felt more exposed and vulnerable than ever. My secret was out. I feared I would never again feel on equal footing with these guys.

"I have epilepsy," I explained, removing my giant glove to reveal the gold MediAlert bracelet I wear. The confession did not fall easily from my lips. It was the first time all year I had admitted it to anyone. It wrenched me back, unwillingly, to reality. I convinced the EMTs that I was in familiar territory and had medication at home. They left me in good hands with my teammates, who hoisted me up and conveyed me into the locker room like royalty, never allowing my feet to touch the ground.

The coach appeared and in a fatherly voice told me that I "scared the hell out of a lot of people out there." A special education teacher by day, he called me the next day to chat and make sure I was OK. I admitted to him that I concealed my condition because I don't like being treated as disabled. I was concerned that people's attitudes toward me would change. When he asked what I had done over the long weekend, I felt my cheeks burn while I cringed at the memory of all the beer I had consumed. I had barely slept at all. It was a situation of my own making.

This event renewed my awareness of how relentless epilepsy could be. Outwardly, even my closest friends did not suspect the vulnerability that lurked beneath the surface. Sure, my seizures can be kept at bay with recurrent medication and good health/life practices. But even though I am considered well-managed, I remain a ticking time bomb that can explode from even the slightest variation in my routine. Defense, cheating, denial. They are all futile. Epilepsy always wins.

I returned to the rink a week later to watch the team play its next game, having been advised to sit out the season in the aftermath of such a major seizure. I was incredibly moved when one of my friends skated out onto the ice wearing my jersey. He scored goal after goal, and each time the scorekeeper announced, "Goal. Number forty-seven. Dodson." It remains, statistically, my best hockey game ever.

Although this seizure was emotionally jarring for me—leaving me reeling with disappointment—at the same time, it probably saved my life. I had deluded myself with "outta sight-outta mind" thinking. I believed I could live a carefree party life in college, free from the isolation and fears I had faced since being diagnosed with epilepsy as a young child. This experience made me see that I can never escape my epilepsy. Whether or not I live seizure-free would largely be a matter of self-control. As is the case with many medical conditions, my lifestyle and routine would forever determine the quality of the life I lead.

That Memorial Day was a wake-up call. I learned that many of my social fears were unfounded. The revelation that I had a hidden condition did not alter the relationships I had with my close friends. And, most importantly, I discovered that the choices I was making—and not my epilepsy—were holding me back in college.

A Camp of Our Own

Until the age of twenty-one, the sum total of my experience with epilepsy was limited to myself. I learned the characteristics of my particular flavor of epilepsy, how to handle it medically and socially, and finally, how to accept it as a permanent fixture in my life. Nonetheless, I was completely ignorant about the larger impact of the disease. I did not know anything about the prevalence of epilepsy in society, the range of experiences that other epilepsy sufferers have, and the resources that are available for children and their families.

Then I went to camp.

During my sophomore year in college the economy collapsed. I returned home to find that summer jobs for college kids had evaporated. Experienced engineers and former bankers were filling the hourly jobs in mall retail stores that typically went to kids on summer break. As a Plan B, I went looking for meaningful volunteer and internship opportunities.

Thanks to my neurologist, I discovered that regional chapters of the Epilepsy Foundation conduct summer camps exclusively for children who have epilepsy. In my area, we had an annual camp held at a traditional campground with cabins and bunk beds. There were fields for sports and a lake for water games. On the surface, this looked like any other summer camp for kids. But here, for one week, the organizers created a specially supervised environment where children with epilepsy would meet, play, do sports, and interact safely while experiencing the joys of a real summer sleep-away camp. I applied as a camp staff volunteer hoping I could give something back while also gaining some valuable leadership cred. I could not have anticipated how the experience would change my life.

During my initial interview, the director described the campers as having mild to severe epilepsy, each suffering from different types of seizures. They considered me a priority hire because of my personal history of seizures, but in reality I had no relevant working knowledge or experience that made me useful. As the first day of camp approached, I got very nervous. The director's description of "brain damage" and "soiled linens" echoed in my brain. It was then I first realized that I had never met another person with epilepsy, nor had I ever witnessed someone else having a seizure. A paralyzing fear grew inside that I could not explain.

Training was extensive. The camp was well-equipped with medical personnel, round-the-clock nursing, and a ratio of one adult for about every two to three campers. We learned basic protocols for how to behave around the campers, legal issues associated with supervising minors, and most importantly, seizure recognition and first aid.

We received a crash course on what epilepsy is from a neurological standpoint, including the many different types of seizures we could expect and what to do when a camper had a seizure. I was surprised to discover that some children had seizures as often as hourly and that some were required to wear safety helmets at all times. Epilepsy among our campers ran the gamut from well-controlled to highly volatile.

Counselor orientation caused me to reflect on my personal journey and my own moments of reckoning. I was attending college. I had grown up playing contact sports. I had a driver's license. I was a normal-pretender, holding the reality of epilepsy at arm's length. I was about to experience full-on epilepsy and how it affected not only these campers but also their families. I was afraid—afraid to discover myself in these children, afraid to acknowledge that I was not normal despite all my efforts to play at normalcy.

And there it was. Could I handle the truth about myself?

On the first morning of camp, I sat at the picnic-style tables under the shelter where meals were served surrounded by the campers in my charge—a group of four boys aged nine, ten, eleven and thirteen. During breakfast, the camp nurse came around in a little golf cart. She carried a tackle box containing rows of small disposable cups. Each contained a customized assortment of pills—appearing much like colorful samples from a candy store. One by one my campers accepted their cups, tipping them into their mouths, familiar as they were with the long-practiced rituals of daily medication. After handing a cup to each boy, the nurse then turned to me and smiled. She handed me a similar cup containing the familiar yellow pentagon-shaped pill that I took at the same time each morning and evening.

The boys stared, a mixture of shock and awe filling their eyes. "You have epilepsy?" one of them asked as I emptied the cup into my mouth and chased it with orange juice. "Yup. Just like you," I answered automatically.

Just. Like. You.

It took a second for the words to sink in and to realize the significance of my reply. Here, among these children, I had finally felt what had been missing my whole life. There was a connection—a kinship even—to these bruised little souls who struggled to keep an even keel against the choppy waves of unpredictable brain synapses. Like me, each of them was isolated in some way by their epilepsy. But here, in this campground, specially outfitted with sympathetic volunteers, unobtrusive medical personnel and stringent safety measures, we were a team, a gang—a band of brothers. Even more importantly, in this moment, epilepsy was the new *normal*.

The campers felt a little more comfortable talking with me than with the other counselor in our cabin, who did not have epilepsy. During meals, we all sat together and they opened up about their conditions, speaking candidly with each other and comparing notes—perhaps for the first time to anyone their age—about the specific attributes of their individual disorders. They were all well-versed in the dos and don'ts, and each knew his own triggers. One child, for example, was exceptionally sensitive to loud noises, while another could drop from the slightest amount of excitement or anxiety. They shared what types of seizures I should expect. One camper warned me privately in a whisper that he would likely pee himself. He brought a supply of pamper-like protectors to keep his bed dry at night.

I stressed over experiencing my first seizure as a spectator. When my friends witnessed my seizures they were quite shaken afterward. I worried that I would be startled myself and unable to respond. In truth, the response for a seizure is simple. There isn't much to do for a person except to keep them safe by moving furniture or objects away from them until the seizure stops. During a seizure, even a small child can seem to possess super-human strength. Any attempt to control their movements can be more dangerous to the person trying to help. Get in their way, and they can kick the teeth right out of your head! A lot of people try to put something in the person's mouth to prevent them from biting their tongue. That's a good way to lose a finger! The single most important thing to do during a seizure is to watch the time. Most seizures last a few seconds or less than a minute and are not harmful. If the seizure does not resolve within five minutes, however, then it's important to call 911, as a prolonged seizure state—known as *status epilepticus*—can cause permanent damage. Paramedics are trained to administer emergency medication in these cases.

I did not have to wait long. I was awkwardly supervising the arts and crafts activities. A little girl was making a necklace for her sister, stringing an infinite numbers of colored beads in no particular pattern. We were having a nice conversation when she suddenly spilled all the beads and dropped to the floor. It was so sudden and terrifying that I forgot everything I had learned and ran frantically to the nearest counselor for help. With complete nonchalance, the counselor said to me, "Relax. She is just having a seizure."

The little girl sure didn't look OK to me. Her eyes became vacant and rolled slightly upward while she vibrated on the floor. She made a strained sound and saliva dripped from her mouth. It seemed like an eternity before she stopped, but in reality it was only about forty seconds. Remarkably, she came to and shook it off, then got back up and finished her necklace while I picked up the beads she spilled. I carry the memory of witnessing this encounter as if it were yesterday.

There was one thing all of these campers had in common. None of them had ever spent a single night away from home, let alone close to a full week. They were very much accustomed to and dependent upon constant interactions with their parents. I heard a lot of "I wish my mom could see me do this," or "I can't wait to tell my dad." Some of the kids had younger or older siblings. It was clear from listening to them talk that their social spheres did not extend much beyond their immediate families.

I wondered how these overburdened families were spending their time while their epilepsy-affected members were safely tucked away at camp. It did not take long for me to recognize that having a child with epilepsy could be taxing upon a family's lifestyle. I thought about my own parents. I realized that I would awaken at night sometimes and find my mother sitting on the side of my bed. I never considered how it came to be that my pill bottles were never empty. Or how it was that my mother would too-often appear on the road while I was walking home from school. Or why my parents allowed me to have my own cell phone before it was commonplace for kids my age.

One of the more surprising revelations for me was how physically delicate these young boys in my charge seemed to be. I hadn't realized how fortunate I was to have been able to perform as an athlete in both baseball and hockey without any limitations. I worked hard at pitching, batting, skating and puck-handling, all of which required significant physical exertion. Several of my campers had limitations on exertion or excitement. They pursued mainly adventures of the mind, either through video games or science-fantasy books. One boy enjoyed writing his own stories and regaled us with his creepy fantasy-fiction in the late-night darkness of our cabin.

Even as I tried to understand the subtleties of each camper's condition, I caught myself making subconscious comparisons to my own condition. My seizures were not as frequent, or my limitations were not as restrictive, or my need for medication was not as great. I admonished myself, hating that I was being judgmental or perhaps unkind to these innocents by trying to discover the line that separated me from them. Indeed, I was very touched by each of them. They begged for stories about playing hockey, about college life at the University of Oregon, and even about girls. They asked a lot of questions about my seizures and how it affected my lifestyle. I looked into their wide-eyed faces and said emphatically, "I have epilepsy. Epilepsy doesn't have me!"

After a lifetime trying to pass myself off as normal, I surprised myself by letting go of the last thread of my self-spun illusion. And this is when my life clicked into place. The more I showed the kids that I was just like them, the more they engaged. The milestones of my life did not divide me from them; they offered hope to these children. I was no longer an authority figure there to barricade them from hazards. I was a leader showing them a way to live with epilepsy.

It can be hard to see that children with epilepsy are far more than a diagnosis and pills. I remembered the dull ache of isolation during my childhood and the frustration I felt at not being able to articulate what I needed. Now I realize that I, we, need a human connection. We need a community that understands, and that fosters understanding. With all the love and good intentions in the world, the people closest to me could not fill the void—simply because they could not experience epilepsy. They could never empathize with the fear of the darkness or the uncertainty of living knowing that a seizure was imminent.

This unexpected moment of clarity proved to be very healing for me. While I could not go back and make my childhood whole, I was now in a position to offer that understanding to others. I was accustomed to insisting, "I don't have it so bad." It was an artifact of my denial. Now, I was eager to show these campers, "I am just like you." By association, perhaps they could grow to be a little like me.

It was so simple. With that acceptance, for the first time, epilepsy brought meaning to my life. Children looked up to me. I could make a difference.

That night the counselors put on a show for the campers. Another counselor and I went through the locker of old costumes and selected a pair of garish pink tutus. With several days' growth of beard on our faces and very much in need of showers, we dressed up as ridiculously ugly women and danced to "I'm a Barbie girl, in a Barbie world!" It was an instant classic to be repeated in future years. I had never been less like myself, and yet I had never felt more comfortable in my own skin.

A Role to Play

By my junior year in college I was well on my way as a sociology major. Sociology is one of those things that cause many people to roll their eyes. "What are you going to do with that?" they ask. "Is that pre-law?" asked a relative, hopefully. I've heard my share of "social science is pseudo-science" cracks.

I was set on the path toward sociology by a favorite high school teacher. She saw the way I agonized over the human condition in her Race Relations class. Was it my experience with epilepsy that made me sensitive to those who are marginalized? I was very inspired to learn about the jagged edges of the real world. My favorite books back then were *Catcher in the Rye* and *A Clockwork Orange*. I loved the opportunity to take a dangerous journey with the characters and not—much to the chagrin of my English teachers—to examine their styles and symbolism.

Sociology fit me to a T, with its opportunity to dive deep into issues such as race and social injustice. I devoured nonfiction accounts of life in ghettos, prisons, and various socioeconomically side-lined populations. The study of society felt like a noble cause—"pre-life," if you will. But it wasn't until that summer of junior year that the sociology lens truly came into focus for me.

I spent that summer engaged in three very different vol-unteer activities. In addition to working at epilepsy camp, where I volunteered for three summers, I also interned at a law firm that did defense work mainly for gang kids. Then I finished out the summer working as a counselor at a youth hockey camp in Minnesota. It was a mind-blowing set of experiences when juxtaposed, honing my skills at supervision, sensitivity, and social engagement.

The camp children with epilepsy had an innocent fra-gility that tugged at my heart. This invisible and poorly understood disease, one I knew only too well, left these children isolated from their peers and local communities. By contrast, the kids who fell into gangs were hardened by low socio-economic conditions and fractured family units, following the dark ways of the lawless young leaders in their neighborhood for survival. I grew up a mere ten miles away, yet kids in these neighborhoods did not see from their vantage point how education and lawfulness offered them any promise of dividends.

Finally, there were the youth hockey players, culti-vated to be unruly and physically violent on the ice. Many of them attended this particular camp as a steppingstone, looking for bigger opportunities with elite leagues that would open the doors to professional careers. In profes-sional hockey, aggressive behavior is not only condoned, but handsomely rewarded and idolized by fans. After bashing each other all day during triple practices, the kids shed their protective layers down to their rambunctious chewy centers. I was the buzzkill counselor tasked with ensuring lights were out by ten.

In the midst of these summer experiences, the universe called out to me in a futuristic dream.

"HEY, LOOK AROUND AND PAY ATTENTION!" it ordered me.

"ARE YOU TALKING TO ME?" I asked.

"YES, NIMROD, I AM TALKING TO YOU!" it answered.

I felt as if suspended at the crossroads of some massive intergalactic cloverleaf. People seemed to whiz by me. I recognized some of my close buddies heading toward careers in business or the sciences. Then, certain highways and byways came into clearer focus before me. I could see the world of epilepsy and our sweet kids' camp bathed in bright summer colors down a small side street. I wept for those children, connected to me by a disease we all dread. Way over there were the would-be gang kids lit in shades of gray, whose highway veered perilously close to my own. The combination of innocence, experience and destiny among these young kids touched my heart. Their exit out of poverty was obstructed by bigger kids, who blinded them with bucks, bullets, and bling. In the distance were the hockey players wrapped in an icy fog, slamming into each other and taking cheap shots, until one by one they dropped through various trap doors, exiting the rink and falling randomly into slow-motion, work-a-day jobs. They would forever dream of the Stanley Cup, eventually laying their crushed NHL dreams at the feet of their own children. Life, I came to realize, is a series of accidents, harsh realizations, and deliberate choices. There, but for the grace of God, go I. This speedbump was my transition to adulthood. It was time to leave my childhood innocence behind and make serious life choices.

Emerging from these cosmic visions and some very real conversations with myself, I discovered a role I could play in this mixed-up world. Empathy is its own skillset, I realized, and I could put my experiences to work as a counselor and advocate. As different as these groups were, all the narratives resonated with me. I felt not only in a unique position to help but also compelled to do so. I wanted to be part of the solution, contributing to the betterment of the world by engaging with troubled youth in a direct and positive way. Drawn to one-on-one interaction, I chose a role that allows me to bring a human touch to those who rarely feel it. And after a lifetime of feeling like I repeatedly missed the mark, I relished the thought of becoming trained and highly competent in these skills. I knew then I was headed toward a career in social services, working with those in society who fall through the cracks.

Studying sociology can be very theoretical and highly quantitative in the context of a liberal arts education. These are not my strong suits. Nonetheless, I muddled through some tough required theory and statistics courses, absorbing enough to thrive when I finally hit the rich assortment of electives. Sure, many people shrug off sociology as an easy major—the courses football players take to maintain academic eligibility. I didn't think there was anything easy about facing the truth about our society. The way in which we impose structures that reinforce differences among colors, classes, and beliefs. The way we reinforce artificial structures to push down others who aren't like us. The way the privileged are oblivious to their privilege. The way some people come into this world with their doom preordained by socioeconomic factors they cannot control. I studied the sociology of families as well as addiction, abuse, and prison culture. I studied mental illness, race and ethnicity, suicide prevention, and poverty.

Through all this academic enlightenment, epilepsy remained both the source of my social anxiety and the inspiration for my studies. When I thought of prejudice, stereotyping and marginalization, I always drew a connection to living with epilepsy. It was not unusual to find epilepsy or disability as a theme in many of my college papers and projects. So while I was busy learning what the university had to teach, I simultaneously found myself on a journey of personal exploration, discovery, and acceptance.

All in the Family

These days, we must choose our words carefully. A person isn't short; they are vertically challenged. Children who fall behind in school may be developmentally challenged. Indeed, my poor, bald-headed grandpa joked that he was "follicly challenged." I ran afoul of this type of challenge-speak when my parents looked into getting me accommodations in school. Epilepsy was a medical diagnosis, we were told, and not a learning or ability "challenge." There was no box for "synapse-challenged" that allowed kids with epilepsy any leeway.

I had mixed feelings about the school-testing and accommodation business. I confess I was reassured when the school said I did not qualify as "disabled" or "having a disability" by virtue of my epilepsy. Nonetheless, the condition clearly hampered my ability to perform in school, such as when taking tests under stress conditions or when called upon to process dozens of multiple-choice questions. As I progressed from high school to college, my uneven performance from class to class challenged me to keep questioning why epilepsy was not recognized as a disability. I continued to ask the difficult questions. Do those of us who suffer with seizure disorders fit the model of other "accepted" disabilities? Should we have access to the types of accommodations to which other outlier students are entitled? Why isn't the fact of epilepsy taken at face value as a learning or performance issue by school counselors and administrators? Is it right that in order to receive accommodations we must be reassessed—a process which I found embarrassing and demoralizing—and assigned to some other approved disability category?

Although it is well beyond my skillset to answer these questions single-handedly, I used the resources and opportunities of my college coursework in sociology to address again and again the issues and challenges that came with having epilepsy. In one particular class, I studied the effect children with disabilities have on families. I very much wanted to study *epilepsy* in families, but unfortunately, there was no available literature on the approved journal list that specifically assessed the burden that a child with epilepsy places on the family unit. It turns out epilepsy is not only invisible in society; it is invisible in social science as well.

In my very unscientific way, I set out instead to see what I could learn from published studies about families that had children with disabilities. I posed the question: to what extent would documented models of families that have a child with disabilities resonate with the realities of growing up with epilepsy? It turns out—to a very great extent!

I feel it is important to explain what I discovered, and will do so in as plain a manner as possible. Much of the social research on families focuses on family structure and variations in "social norms" that affect family structure, such as marital status, same-sex parents, interracial couples, and socioeconomic status. These studies look at whether family structure affects the well-being of children within the family. My question worked in the opposite direction. When a family has a child who is impaired by disability, how does it affect the other individuals within the family, family stability, and socioeconomic status?

Of course, impairments among disabled children vary greatly. Most research I found aggregates "disabled child" into a single category defined as any child who has an identified impairment, whether the cause is medical, physical, learning, or mental, and where the impairment requires things such as continued medical care, therapy, education, developmental support, or other interventions. The terms *impairment* and *disability* are often used interchangeably, although some scholars like to differentiate between these terms, or prefer one term over the other. Epilepsy is a very broad category, and can cause children to have any or all of the factors used to define impairment or disability. A child with epilepsy can range from well-controlled on medication with no other issues, to having an array of physical, learning, and developmental challenges—sometimes severe, or anywhere in between.

Children with disabilities have special needs that require a greater level of attention, support, and resources from parents than other children. The parental duties related to a disabled child are in addition to all the other basic and traditional functions found within the family. Disabilities are often discovered at birth or at a very young age, and impaired children tend to remain within the family longer than non-impaired children. Because of these and other considerations, families with children who have disabilities experience family-hood differently than other families where disabilities are not present.[1]

One sociologist describes the family as having both public and private dynamics. Privately, a family grows into a routine of love and support for its members. Publicly, a family assumes the mantle placed on it by society.[2] When a disability is present in the family, it taxes the family on both fronts. Families that care for a child with epilepsy— like those with other disabilities—face stresses that not only impact the private life of the family, but also compromise the way the family interacts publicly with, and is accepted by, the community. I remember the public exposure my on-ice seizure event received and how quickly rumors and false information spread around the neighborhood. People approached me with downward glances. My hockey coach was reluctant to let me play. Although I was no different than the person I was a week earlier, my experience in the community changed dramatically.

Epilepsy retains several social stigmas, born out of ignorance, that often invoke unintentional insensitivity from others. I've seen more than one television show that used epilepsy—jokingly—as a metaphor for awkwardness or freakishness. In that light, imagine the difficulties families face when they must disclose their child's risks and emergency seizure procedures when interacting with other families, friends, or schools. Every time my family brought in a new babysitter, or if I was invited to sleep over at a friend's house, there was a litany of facts, procedures,

---

1 Janice McLaughlin, Dan Goodley, Emma Clavering, Pamela Fisher. *Families Raising Disabled Children: Enabling Care and Social Justice*, Palgrave MacMillan, 2008.

2 Cherlin, Andrew. *Public and Private Families: An Introduction* 7th Edition. McGraw-Hill Education, 2012.

and protocols that my mother ran through in the event I experienced a seizure. It all sounded pretty scary to me. Put him on the floor. Move the furniture away from him. Do not put anything in his mouth—especially your own fingers. Call 9-1-1.

Even the ability to enjoy a family outing, such as a movie, concert or sporting event can be hindered by the stress of encountering unexpected triggers for seizures. I remember being around seven years old when my family attended a performance of Riverdance. At one point in the show, without prior warning, they used very bright flashing red lights on stage. My mother sat with her hands over my eyes until the unexpected encounter with this classic epilepsy trigger subsided.

Given the sensitivity society has toward "labels," social scientists take care to describe and compare norms without seeming to label and stigmatize their subjects. They do this by offering more precise distinctions in terminology. One group, for example, suggests using the term "impairment" only when a limitation is experienced personally, such as lacking a limb or having a defective learning mechanism. They reserve the term "disability" to describe when society excludes or limits individuals with impairments. To follow this logic, disability is less about an individual's physical state. Instead, we look to society to better accommodate the wide variation among human abilities. [1]

Since epilepsy is most commonly seen as a medical condition rather than either an impairment or a disability, it is no surprise that society does a poor job of addressing the needs of those who are afflicted. For example, parking, seating and access for the wheelchair-bound have been in common practice for decades, mandated by

1   McLaughlin et al.

law to be incorporated into all public buildings. By contrast, a person with epilepsy lives in a world of traps and triggers, never knowing when the screaming red lights of an ambulance will speed by, or a dance floor in a bar or restaurant will switch on strobing lights. Movies present vivid hazards without warning, blind to the dangers posed by extreme sound and light special effects. Only recently, when the intense action sequences in Disney's *Incredibles 2* movie triggered seizures in many young viewers around the country, was a seizure warning finally added to posters and trailers.

I also discovered data that suggest families that have children with disabilities experience inequalities that families with children without disabilities do not. When children have disabilities, the family often suffers as a whole from unequal opportunities and outcomes, including financial hardship, stress and anxiety resulting from social barriers, prejudices, and poor access to services. However, researchers wish us to consider that it is not the impairment of the child that threatens the quality of family life with distress and hardship. They fault the structures, systems, policies and attitudes of society toward the family for failure to accommodate outliers. It's not that "a child with disabilities disables the whole family." Rather, "the child does not handicap the family—society does."[1]

This idea that society disables the entire family is borne out by a comprehensive study performed between 1985 and 1988 in the United Kingdom. Researchers found that 75 percent of parents with a disabled child did not

---

1 Monica Dowling and Linda Dolin. "Families with Children with Disabilities—Inequalities and the Social Model," *Disability and Society*, Vol 16, No. 1, 2001, pp. 21.

have enough money to care for their child, parents of disabled children had lower incomes, and mothers of disabled children were less likely to be employed. These characteristics also meant there is greater anxiety or stress day-to-day as well as limited access to resources such as childcare or domestic help. Furthermore, they reported a strong relationship between disability and household income: areas with higher poverty had higher rates of disability.[1]

I met an extraordinary family that had two children, fraternal twin brother and sister, both of whom had epilepsy. The children required six different medications multiple times per day. To put this in perspective, the retail cost of my single twice-daily pill is about $5,000 per year. The financial demands of epilepsy outstripped this family's ability to do much more than manage the demands of their children's medical condition. Epilepsy plunged them into debt. The last I heard they were in danger of losing their home.

Families that deal with epilepsy face stress from many fronts, not just financial. Dealing with both the paperwork of medical coverage and the need to repeat the family's story again and again to healthcare workers, teachers, and babysitters are punishing to both parent and child. The constant stream of appointments with doctors, counselors, and labs involve significant travel and waiting time. These activities are not easily accommodated into rigid work schedules or school routines. Often, one parent is forced to give up a full-time job in order to function as general manager for the child's care. A friend of my mother's, whose daughter's epilepsy caused the child to fall behind in school, was forced to leave a lucrative full-time job and adapt to at-home self-employment projects

---

1   Ibid.

in order to maintain the flexibility she required to meet the increasing demands of her daughter's care.

Within the family, the mother is most often the person tasked as primary caregiver and advocate for the child with a disability. I saw this time and time again when meeting youths with epilepsy. Almost exclusively, the mother was charged with managing the complexity and demands of her child's life with epilepsy. One summer at camp, I had primary responsibility for three young boys in my cabin. I also had three other counselors who assisted me. I cannot overstate this point: it took four counselors to manage the needs of three children with epilepsy!

It was eye-opening to experience what it was like to be on the "other side"—to be the caregiver rather than the cared-for. Naively, I had brought my laptop to camp, figuring I could check emails or watch movies after bedtime. Silly me! There was no off-duty time—not even after dark. Caring for my charges proved to be a 24/7 activity. None of the kids had ever spent a night outside their own homes; they each faced separation anxiety. One boy soiled his linens many times per night. (Guess who got to change them?) To make things worse, we were facing a string of violent, late-summer thunderstorms. One of my boys was extremely photosensitive, which meant the lightning that accompanied violent summer storms, particularly in the dark of night, added to his already inevitable chance of seizures.

My young campers represented a range of circumstances. One was a nine-year old. He was an only child and attended public school. His epilepsy required four different medications taken three times daily. One of these medications gave him ADHD-like symptoms which, in turn, affected his behavior and performance in school. Although he was grade appropriate in school for his age, he was nonetheless on an Individual Educational Plan

(IEP) that provided him with extra time to complete tests and with special assistance both inside and outside the classroom. I want to emphasize that his accommodations in school were for ADHD, which was an effect of his medication, and not for epilepsy. In his case, his seizures were primarily nocturnal.

Another boy, who was ten years old, was one of the brightest children I have ever met. He was clearly intellectually gifted, and his knowledge seemed mainly self-taught. He and his older sister both had epilepsy. This young guy would speak to me about any subject from science to science fiction, but he refused to discuss epilepsy at all. I learned that his family was struggling to keep a roof over their heads largely because of the cost of managing epilepsy for two children. Other family members were stepping in to provide a financial safety net for them which, in itself, was affecting the parents' self-esteem and causing a tremendous burden of guilt on the children. The children's attendance at camp was a gift from their grandmother. It served to give a new opportunity to the children as well as a well-deserved respite for their parents.

My final camper was an eight-year-old. He had a severe type of epilepsy that affected his mental capacity to the point that he functioned at the level of a pre-schooler. He was sweet and shy, but unable to share much about himself. For example, he knew what state he lived in but not the name of the town. This boy was on a Ketogenic diet, an extreme and sometimes controversial treatment for children with severe forms of epilepsy. Ketogenic diets are high in fat and proportionally low in carbohydrates—similar to the Atkin's diet, but far more restrictive—keeping the body in a persistent state of ketosis. Ketogenic diets have been shown effective in helping people with severe epilepsy for whom available medications fail to control seizures.

This little guy came to camp with a cooler full of individually portioned-out meals that he was to eat instead of the camp's food. The combination of his medicine and strict diet caused him to vomit regularly. Due to his diet's lack of carbohydrates he was not particularly active, causing him to nap several times throughout the day.

Together, my research on families and my volunteer experiences opened my eyes to several important things about epilepsy. While epilepsy is regarded more as a medical condition than a disability, a family where a child has epilepsy shares many key characteristics with studied models of families with impaired or disabled children. In my discussions with epilepsy families, children with epilepsy impose comparable burdens on families, both privately and publicly, compared to families whose children have other types of disabilities. Furthermore, I found society at large to be somewhat blind and tone-deaf to the needs of people with epilepsy within the conventional spectrum of accommodated, differently abled citizens.

There is a reason I took the time to study this issue and to discuss it here. While society has improved the conditions for people with many types of impairments and disabilities worldwide, it has yet to meet this same standard with the epilepsy population. There needs to be a greater understanding of how society can accommodate children with seizure disorders in mainstream educational programs and in public places. Teachers, coaches, daycare workers, and administrators—to name just a few—need better education about the effects of epilepsy on children and their families. In particular, families who are already overburdened managing epilepsy should not be forced to jump through additional diagnostic hoops in order to squeeze their child into alternative, pre-defined, "acceptable" categories of disability for which school services and accommodations are readily offered to others. As a high schooler, I found my counselors wholly unprepared and uninterested in addressing epilepsy-related learning and performance issues. I am just guessing that as I get older and experience different types of workplaces and work conditions, I will find similar speedbumps in the adult world of epilepsy.

Stigmatism

I must confess that it has taken me years to progress from the initial enthusiasm at telling my stories, to waxing and waning interest in writing this book, to various times where the end was clearly in sight. The longer I put off finishing, the more of my story there was to tell. Since starting to record my tales, I have graduated from college, faced the shocking realities of surviving in the real world as an adult, entered the workforce, married my best friend, bought a home, and now I have a new-born child. Ever persistent, life happens.

Doctors commonly tell parents of children with epilepsy to reset their expectations. I was not aware of this as a child; my parents have only recently confessed this to me. It is hard to generalize about the effects of a disease for which the experience is so variable and individualized. For every story like mine there are thousands of others with different sorts of outcomes. Epilepsy alters many of life's trajectories. As a group, we are less likely to excel and achieve in higher education, we have greater difficulty maintaining relationships, and we are disqualified—because of inherent dangers while climbing, driving, or operating heavy machinery—from pursuing many vocational or career options. My relative good fortune is not wasted on me. I cherish my life every day as the miracle it is.

I often think back to those times when I was privately devastated by the successive "a-ha" revelations of living with a chronic disease. As life-altering and life-defining as those moments seemed at the time, they nonetheless pale by comparison to the horrors I found in the real world—the struggle to make a living, to pay the rent, and to figure out where each next meal would come from. There was no time or energy for self-pity. Though ever-present, epilepsy got pushed to the background as I encountered a million new fears. How would I go about establishing a sustainable routine—to "design," in essence, what would become my life? And even if I were able to cobble together a balanced existence, what guarantee did I have that the choices I made would continue to be available to me? Life carries a lot of uncontrollable variables such as health insurance policy, military draft laws, the economy, unpredictable natural disasters, just to name a few. As of this writing, my epilepsy brothers and sisters across the U.S. remain on tender hooks as to whether our federal government will abolish health legislation that today guarantees insurance coverage for pre-existing conditions.

Fortunately, life has a way of working out. I look back now and cannot believe I endured the transition from college to full-time employment. My first job out of college was as a counselor at a highly intense halfway house. I worked from 2:00 p.m. to 10:00 p.m., and my "weekend" days off were Tuesday and Wednesday. My clients were drug-addicted felons between the ages of sixteen and twenty-five who were either on the progression from prison to parole or under court-order as an alternative to incarceration. They had seen and lived through horrors much worse than the secrets I carried around with me. Many had already faced down death, whether by illegal substance or weapon, on more than one occasion. More than a few had not had parental contact or support in years.

Entering their world upended all my past fears and trepidations. I felt a twinge of guilt for the familial safety net I've always had around me. In this setting, having a cushy life was the stigma. I disguised my "silver spoon" upbringing in much the same way as I had learned to disguise my epilepsy. To reveal it or to be "outed" would threaten my credibility among the hardened residents. Success on the job depended upon my ability to wrap empathy with authority.

Although epilepsy had always been my kryptonite, in this setting it was my superpower. I was well trained at compartmentalizing and toggling between my private and public faces. In the way I once masked my fears, I shrouded my background from view. I assumed the façade of street-smart authority and wore it with confidence. It helped that I believed in my job. The tough love I delivered was truly in the best interest of these unfortunate and misguided young men.

Working in social services and corrections is challenging and often heartbreaking. While most of us rely on a circle of family and friends, my clients had been betrayed or neglected by nearly every relation. To these young men, the "system" was faceless and dispassionate. There were no rewards, no upsides, no security, and no permanence. They adapted to life like animals in the wild—their ears always listening and their nerve endings always primed to run or pounce. My efforts to counsel or support them were processed through a jaded filter. They trusted no one and tested me and my limits constantly.

One refrain that I heard a lot was, "You just don't understand." Those words were familiar to me. They had been my knee-jerk defense mechanism, often uttered in self-pity. How weird to hear those very words shoved back in my face! Isolation can create an emotional vacuum, but it can sometimes be a safe space. As long as you believe that no one understands what you are going through, you give yourself permission to be miserable. In the case of these kids, their misery was an invitation to retreat into drugs, crime, and other forms of social disobedience.

I surprised myself by finding resonance between living with epilepsy and falling into a life of crime. Obstacles are obstacles. I think innate survivors recognize each other in the wild. Just as there is honor among thieves, I believe there is empathy among survivors. My go-to stance for calming a raging resident in our facility was a quiet, neutral stare. I would look deep into their eyes, searching for the pain I knew was there, and then looking far beyond that for the lost innocence. In that moment, if they were looking back, they could see beyond my own compartment of authority and recognize the shadows of the scared and angry child I once was.

Finding that connection in my emotional memory banks was empowering for me in this setting. It helped me to momentarily disrupt the cycle of anger and distrust with these hardened teens, creating an opening in which to be instructive or therapeutic. "These rules and I are here to help you achieve your goals," I would repeat, just as I was trained. It worked in many cases, but it was also a double-edged sword. Sensing I was their advocate as opposed to their warden, many of these kids would turn on a dime and begin looking for exceptions and allowances: an extension to curfew, a quick unauthorized phone call, or a few bucks. They were well-practiced in the con, living for the shortcuts and quick fixes. It's part of their disease.

This experience was a moment of transformation for me. It's when I first became aware that my past with epilepsy could pay dividends—endowing me with skills that could be useful in a professional setting. Sure, I could not relate to being a felon or an addict, but I did have empathy for those whose lives had been hijacked by powers beyond their control. It was helpful to be able to understand that one's lot in life is only partially hindered by the labels and stigmas attached by society. In the end, whether it was advice to the young men in my charge or a prescription for my own destiny, I saw that empowerment, independence, and success come only from the choices we make for ourselves.

Vive La Différence

I first encountered this expression—vive la différence—during my many years of studying
French language. It translates roughly to
"long live the difference." Oddly, it seems to
have no identifiable French or literary origin.
As far as I can tell, and through the magic of
Google, Spencer Tracy first proclaimed this to
Katherine Hepburn in the 1949 film *Adam's
Rib*. A talented female lawyer, she argued to her
nemesis that they were equal in every sense,
while Tracy's character was distracted by the
female attributes of his beautiful co-star. He
was grateful for that little difference.

This expression is not only used convey
this somewhat out-of-date and arguably
sexist message. For many years, the
French-speaking island country of Haiti
used "Vive La Différence" as its tourism
tag line. Here, it encouraged world trav-
elers to embrace Haiti for its uniqueness
as a vacation destination. It is a plea to
appreciate the beauty of its diversity.

Growing up with health differences, learning this beautiful battle cry was an antidote for my self-pity doldrums. It brought meaning to something my mother used to tell me about my epilepsy. "Everyone has a certain baggage that they carry," she said. "This is yours." So I paid particular attention to the people around me, not so much to document how I was different, but rather to discover the ways each of us is unique.

There was the girl who sat in front of me in one of my classes. She was tall and beautiful—and perhaps a little out of my league. I liked to look at her beautiful hair and imagine running my fingers through it. She was an excellent student and a talented athlete. I noticed she would sometimes reach under her sweater and feel for the small object that was clipped to the top of her leggings. I assumed this was her cellphone, as we were not allowed to have them visible during school hours. But one day I saw her open this gadget and push some buttons. It was not a phone at all. It was an insulin pump! Somewhere she had a narrow catheter inserted into her stomach that was regulating her insulin as her blood sugar rose and fell. I never found the courage to ask her about it. Or more precisely, my own experience warned me that to ask might violate her privacy or embarrass her. I wondered if she felt broken the way I did. I imagined her as a small girl, having to endure repeated insulin injections. Compared to her baggage, my childhood monthly blood tests no longer seemed such a high price to pay.

My sister had a friend who was born with just one fully formed arm. I met her several times before I became aware of what I immediately termed her missing arm. But my first impression was wrong. To this young woman's credit, she was not "missing" anything. She had what she had and she made the best of it. She became a competitive fencer and excelled at it, finding in this one-armed sport a perfect fit for the person she is.

I know at least two guys who were diagnosed with testicular cancer young in life. I put myself through the mental exercise of being examined, enduring diagnostic tests, and then finally being given the news of the radical surgery that would necessarily follow. There was no privacy at all for these guys. Everyone in their neighborhoods knew their business and the resulting personal loss that followed. But to them, they felt lucky to have been diagnosed early and to have been treated in a way that left them healthy and cancer-free.

Another guy had a large birthmark on his face. It was a congenital anomaly commonly called a "port wine stain"—a large red patch over nearly half of his face. Caused by a vascular malformation beneath the surface of the skin, this mark left my buddy looking a little bit like the Phantom of the Opera. In every other way this kid was healthy and vital, but his unique face mask could be off-putting to potential friends. I noticed that he was shy, particularly around girls. It was odd how people treated him—callous and mean, all because of something that affected nothing but the color of a small area of skin. I tried to imagine how he felt when he looked in the mirror each day. Did he see his red mark as disguising his true self? Did he see himself without the mark? Or was the mark something he accepted as uniquely and truly his? A divine gift, perhaps, that defined him or endowed him with special powers?

Another classmate of mine was confined to a wheelchair from a very young age. He had a physical developmental anomaly that made him very small and left his bones especially brittle. His physical impairment was severe enough that he required assistance in school at all times, as he lacked the strength even to hold a book or to write. Nonetheless, he was remarkably socialized with our group. He had a great sense of humor and was very interactive verbally during lunch and recess. Unbeknownst to us, he spent months exercising and practicing in order to be able to stand with the rest of us at graduation. We were all in tears as he took his victory walk across the stage—assisted by a walker—to receive his diploma on his own two feet. I think about this guy often—how the mobility that so many of us take for granted was for him the crowning achievement of that milestone day.

A friend of my sister's was struck suddenly with a disease to her eyes. Over a period of just months her vision diminished to about 10 percent, leaving her legally blind with only marginal peripheral vision. She was a top student and a talented athlete. Although her life plan was suddenly and irrevocably altered, she strived to maintain as much normalcy as possible with incredible support from her parents and siblings. To her credit, she continued to figure skate competitively, graduated high school, then went away to college—eventually earning a Master's Degree in counseling.

Throughout this book I have tried to tell a story of discovery, of self-realization, of overcoming obstacles, and of personal triumph. But for every success story and upbeat anecdote there are scores of children who remain debilitated by injury or disease. I don't in any way mean to minimize the challenges these children and their families face. Not every story has a fairy tale ending.

What I have learned, however, (and it took me a very long time to get there) is that others do not define our success. We do a disservice to ourselves to allow broad, common yardsticks, such as SAT scores, grades, sports, earnings, and job titles, to determine whether or not we are successful. Some milestones are measured in smaller strokes. Others achievements stand on their own and cannot be compared.

My mother claims that she always knew I would grow up to be a social worker. Not because some assessment or aptitude guidelines pigeon-holed me into this career. Rather, she saw from an early age my compassion for those less fortunate and my desire to repair what I could manage from my little corner of the world. I will never be a wealthy investment banker or play on a Stanley Cup team. But I am excellent at a profession that can, literally, change the outcomes of the lives of victimized kids—kids whose only wrong turn in life was being born to the wrong parents. If I cannot cure epilepsy, at least I can make a difference in the lives of these kids, who are no less victims of their circumstances than I am of mine. Through this strange confluence of self-discovery and my battle with epilepsy, I have found myself and my purpose.

Taking Charge

T here are so many types of seizure disorders that encompass the disease known as
epilepsy. As a result, there is also a broad
spectrum of affectedness. Tragically, some
children with epilepsy are very debilitated by
their condition and require heightened levels
of care or specialized living environments into
adulthood. Most sufferers of epilepsy find that
managing their symptoms runs the gamut
from chronic ailment to constant annoyance.
Some expect seizures many times per day.
Others, like me, have seizures less frequently
or even rarely, yet live in constant fear of that
next occurrence.

Living with epilepsy means living
on medication. Epilepsy drugs have
evolved greatly, even in my own lifetime. Thanks to good science, doctors
now have a broad menu of medications
to prescribe that map to the many different types of seizure disorders. In almost
every case, physicians strive for a balance

between calming the electrical activity of the brain and maintaining the conscious, productive enterprise of the patient. Oftentimes, drugs are added to the mix to mitigate symptoms rather than replacing what is already being taken. This is because patients with epilepsy can be sensitive to changes in medications.

In my experience, taking charge of my life meant learning to take charge of my epilepsy. This included learning all I could about the disease itself. How is epilepsy diagnosed? What is my own personal flavor of epilepsy? What are my most likely triggers? What are the restrictions and warnings specific to my medication regimen? And most importantly, what are the behaviors and actions that are non-negotiable in maintaining my health?

Looking back, I believe it took me three major leaps to achieve what I consider to be true independence as an adult with epilepsy. The first leap was making the transition from living at home with my parents to living independently on the other side of the country as a college student. The second leap was after graduating, when I began to live and work on my own, supporting myself on the strict budget of my meager paycheck. The final leap was coming to terms with my adult goals of being a professional, a husband, and a father. In each case, I was forced to prioritize my wants and needs, make tough choices between fun and necessity, and accept that there would always be a connection between managing my epilepsy and living my life.

One of the first lessons I learned was the importance of understanding how health insurance works and where it comes from. Currently, the law allows children to stay on their parents' health insurance until they turn twenty-six. This can be a ticking time bomb for some. For me, I was very conscious of approaching the age-out deadline.

If I had not found a job with insurance benefits, I would have had to purchase insurance through a state marketplace and absorb that cost into my budget. No one with epilepsy should ever be without health insurance.

Currently, the Affordable Care Act protects people from being denied coverage for pre-existing conditions. However, the legislature continues to flirt with the idea of repealing this provision. A pre-existing condition is the previous documented treatment of a chronic ailment at the time you enroll for coverage. If you maintain continuity of health insurance coverage—which means never being without insurance for even a day—the fact that you have epilepsy rolls over from health plan to health plan and is accepted as a pre-existing condition. But if you allow yourself a lapse in coverage for a period of time, you might find benefits related to epilepsy care will not be allowed if mandatory coverage for pre-existing conditions is struck down.

For generations, health insurance coverage for patients with epilepsy was not in question. In fact, Medicare, which is best known for providing health insurance for Americans over the age of sixty-five, also extends benefits to those of all ages who are considered disabled by epilepsy. But with "entitlement" programs under siege in the legislature, benefits we rely upon today can be wiped away with the stroke of a pen. It is important to know the facts of federal and state health care laws, particularly as they relate to pre-existing conditions. It is also important to be involved with your local chapter of the Epilepsy Foundation, and to help support its lobbying efforts on behalf of people with epilepsy.

Another important learning curve for me related to my prescription medication. There are important considerations that could have serious consequences for my health. My primary medication, Lamictal, has a life-threatening side effect if it is ramped up or tapered off too quickly. For this reason, it is essential that I take my medications on a strict schedule and do not suddenly stop taking it. I have heard of people who, either because they feel fine, they do not like the way they feel on their medications, or cannot afford their prescriptions, decide to stop on their own. A cavalier attitude toward my medications could cost me my life! Anti-seizure drugs and other supplemental drugs that epilepsy patients may take to mitigate side effects are carefully balanced and monitored by your doctor. While it is important to understand the quirks of your particular drugs, never assume that you know enough to self-medicate or self-modulate.

You should also be aware that the law allows pharmacies to substitute generic drugs for name-brand drugs when they are available unless your doctor specifically requests the name brand. There are many reasons why your doctor may request a name-brand drug, including scientific or anecdotal evidence on the effectiveness of the drug. If a generic is available, your doctor may need to complete extra paperwork to get approval for a brand-name drug from your insurance company. However, even if your insurance company approves the dispensing of a more expensive name-brand medication, they still may only pay as much as the less expensive generic, leaving you to pay the rest.

This happened to me when Lamictal's patent ran out and generic substitutes hit the market. I brought the issue back to my doctor. It turns out that there is a chance of variability as you go from brand name to generic. There is also variability between a single drug agent manufactured by different generic suppliers. My doctor felt it was important for me to maintain as consistent a level of medicine in my system as possible. The name brand was the only way, she felt, to ensure that this happened. However, she was willing to let me migrate to the generic drug, if I followed a three-week protocol that would minimize the risks of any sharp drop or spike in medication differences.

I talked to my pharmacist and the situation became even more complex. I discovered that while pharmacists are required to dispense generics unless instructed not to by the physician, their supplying formularies may change generic suppliers at will and without notifying the patient, if and when they find alternative generic sources at lower costs. This means any time the source of generic drug changes, I face the same risks going from generic to generic as changing from name brand to generic. Working in col-laboration with my physician and my pharmacist we came up with a plan. The pharmacist flagged my account with an alert to notify me when the generic source changes. He also showed me where on the pill bottle the name of the generic manufacturer is identified. Each time I get a refill, I check my old bottle against the new one to see if the source changed. If I encounter a change in generic source, I implement my doctor's change-over protocol, which amounts to alternating pills between bottles over two to three weeks to smooth out any differences over an extended timeframe.

I mention these issues to underscore the fact that despite my ability to grow into my epilepsy, to accept it as a lifelong companion, and to learn to live without fear or stigma, there are still a host of outside forces that can change life on a dime for people with epilepsy. To the extent possible, learning about the law, particularly how it relates to healthcare access and health insurance, has become important to my own sense of well-being. As invisible as we are in society, I feel strongly that we must leverage the power of our numbers and learn to speak with one voice. Once I reached voting age, I made it my business to vote for candidates who are unflinching in their support of access to care and coverage for pre-existing conditions.

Finally, I cannot say enough about the Epilepsy Foundation and the committed staff and volunteers at the regional chapters. Not only are the websites a tremendous source of information on local events and national issues, but I credit the community service programs in which I participated with helping to expand my education about my disease, to making visible the invisible community of epilepsy brothers and sisters, and to helping me find my voice as an advocate.

In many ways, pulling together my stories was an exercise in building perspective and making myself whole. If you found this collection of tales entertaining, I am humbled. If these pages help to quash fears or inspire independence, then I am rewarded. Remember, speedbumps can occur anytime and anywhere in life. Take them at your own speed and you will keep moving forward.

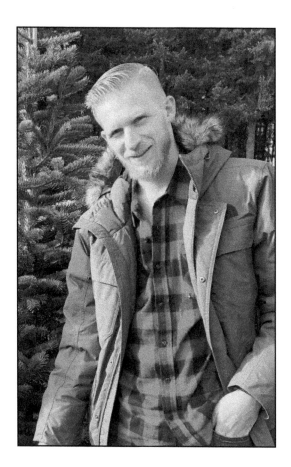

Jonathan Dodson was diagnosed with pediatric absence seizures at the age of four and had his first tonic-clonic seizure in high school while playing hockey. Raised in the Boston suburbs, Dodson is a direct descendant of Oregon Trail pioneers. He holds a BA in sociology from the University of Oregon and lives in Oregon with his wife and young son, where he works as a case worker for Child Protective Services.

CPSIA information can be obtained
at www.ICGtesting.com
Printed in the USA
LVHW041954291119
638856LV00011B/739/P

9 781629 016115